MEDICAL INTERVIEWS

A comprehensive guide to
CT, ST & Registrar
interview skills

Over 120 medical interview questions, techniques and NHS topics explained

3rd Edition

Written by:
Olivier Picard BSc (Hons) MSc

Edited by:
Dan Wood PhD FRCS(Urol)
Consultant Urological Surgeon

Sebastian Yuen MBBS DCH MRCPCH FHEA
Consultant Paediatrician

1

Published by ISC Medical
Tel: 0845 226 9487 – Email: enquiries@iscmedical.co.uk

Third Edition (Revised)
ISBN13: 978-1-905812-24-0

Printed: August 2019

A catalogue record for this book is available from the British Library.

Printed in the United Kingdom by:
Optichrome, Maybury Road, Woking, Surrey GU21 5HX

The author and the editors have, as far as possible, taken care to ensure that the
information given in this text is accurate and up to date at time of publication. The
information within this text is intended as a revision aid for the purpose of the medical interviews. It is not intended, nor should it be used, as a medical reference for
the management of patients or their conditions. Readers are strongly advised to
confirm that the information with regards to specific patient management complies
with current legislation, guidelines and local protocols.

Contents

Preface

Over the past few years, medical interviews have become increasingly competitive. This is especially true for entry into core training (CT) or specialist training (ST). In addition, the interview process itself has become more arduous, with the traditional "sophisticated chat" in front of a panel being replaced by a rotation between a wide range of stations, with often strict marking schedules and limited time to answer. With systematic preparation, everyone can do very well. However, achieving the success you seek will require a number of conditions to be fulfilled:

Know yourself well

Before you can convince a stranger that you are the candidate that they are looking for, it makes sense to convince yourself. An interview is as much about making bold claims such as "I am a good doctor" as it is about proving it with facts. The truth is that most candidates have not really thought about what they can offer; as a result, they often come unstuck when asked for evidence to support their claims.

One student once asked me how she should answer "Why do you want to train in chemical pathology?" I asked her why she was interested in chemical pathology, to which she replied that she did not know. Somehow, she felt that there was a "miracle answer" which would guarantee her the job and that, if she mentioned three reasons fed to her, she could make it. An interview is *your* personal story, *your* experience, strengths and weaknesses; it is not about regurgitating a ready-made answer. So, you must give yourself time to brainstorm your skills and experience. Throughout this book, I will show you how you can achieve this.

Learn, understand and apply key communication frameworks

A relatively small part of the interview process is about knowledge – in some interviews, clinical or factual knowledge is not tested at all. Interviews are mostly a communication exercise where you are expected to demonstrate your suitability in a mature, enthusiastic and confident manner. To achieve this painlessly, you must acquire a good understanding of some of the fundamental pillars of communication. Like the mental or paper-based frameworks and checklists that you use when you take a history from a patient or perform a procedure, there are techniques you acquire and can use and adapt to your circumstances in order to build confident interview answers.

Throughout this book I will show you how to apply a wide range of techniques to structure your answers and illustrate them with personal examples. By applying these techniques to your personal skills, experience and opinions, you will be able to present powerful and confident answers, whilst at the same time remaining (or appearing) spontaneous.

4

Practise, practise, practise

I often compare the preparation for an interview to the preparation that comedians or politicians must go through for a new routine or speech. Although everything they say sounds off-the-cuff, it has been carefully thought through and practised. Good interview candidates sound genuine, unrehearsed and enthusiastic; but, although for some lucky individuals this comes naturally, many will have spent time practising and refining their content and technique. This book will show you how to prepare effectively, whether you are one day, one month or further away from your interview date.

By reading the book, you will quickly come to the realisation that, although you could be asked hundreds of questions, you will always get back to the same handful of themes and communication techniques. It is therefore crucial that you do not try to learn answers to each individual question but, instead, that you concentrate on developing good overall personal knowledge of the topics that are being addressed and of the techniques needed to organise and illustrate your answer. This will give you greater flexibility and a definite ability to cope with pretty much any question.

Good luck with your preparation.

Olivier Picard

How to use this book

This book has been written in a modular fashion so that you can read it in many different ways:

If you have plenty of time to prepare

If you have time, you may wish to read the book once from cover to cover to get a general feel for the techniques used, before going over each section systematically. Interview preparation can be quite intense, particularly if you have a long way to go. Brainstorming, structuring and delivering answers can be tiring if you do too much in one go; so ideally you should take on one section at a time so that you have time to assimilate the information, work on it, practise and refine your approach.

If you are pressed for time or if your interview is imminent

If you are under pressure, or simply too busy to spend much time preparing, you may wish to read the section on key interview techniques first and then select ten to twenty key questions to work on before the interview, spanning a range of topics. It is best to spend quality time (i.e. 5-10 minutes each) preparing a limited number of questions than to prepare hundreds of questions at a rate of 5 seconds per question. At the interview, you will have to make 2 minutes out of your 5 seconds of preparation and the result could prove quite painful (i.e. you will either freeze or start waffling to buy time). It is all about technique and quality rather than quantity. This modular approach enables you to prepare effectively whether you have an interview tomorrow, next week or in a few months' time.

Health warning

In this book, I have provided examples of good and bad answers. Their purpose is to give you an appreciation of what sounds good and bad and how answers can be improved so that you can apply a similar thinking process to your own answers. There are many types of bad answers but there are also many types of good answers. The examples in this book should be taken as illustrations of the techniques discussed and not as a blanket template for all your answers. Instead of trying to replicate each answer faithfully, try to use it to understand each of the principles outlined and to determine how you can then apply these principles to your own situation.

Every candidate is unique and it is pretty much impossible to provide examples that are suitable for all candidates in every specialty. Whenever possible, I have explained how the content can be adapted to the various specialties. What is important is that you understand the techniques and mode of thinking behind the answer so that you can adapt them to your own specialty and circumstances.

THE
SELECTION
PROCESS

1 Structure of the interview

The structure of the interview varies with each deanery[1] and specialty. Interviews typically consist of a succession of 10-minute sessions at three or four stations, each dealing with different topics. There are variations: some interviews have fewer stations, with more time spent at each; other deaneries have more (up to six). A few have kept the old interview format, i.e. a 30- to 45-minute interview with only one panel. In addition, some specialties/deaneries are very strict on time whilst others are less rigid.

Before attending your interview, make sure that you know the format adopted for your specialty in that deanery – this will influence the way in which you will need to respond. If the interviewers are allowing 10 minutes for five questions, including the time that it takes to ask the question, then you know that you must provide answers that fit within a 90-second timeframe. This means that you must be more regimented and concise in order not to exceed your time.

The stations used at interview can be split between:

- Formal stations (i.e. those designed as a traditional, formal question and answer session); and

- Practical stations (i.e. those which require a more hands-on approach from the candidate – including role play or clinical skills).

On the next few pages, I have set out the different types of stations that you can expect to meet at your interview.

---

[1] See full list in chapter 19

1.1 Formal interview stations

Formal interview stations comprise two or three interviewers asking pre-determined questions of a candidate and scoring the responses. The stations below are those that are commonly found at CT and ST/ Registrar levels.

Portfolio station
The portfolio station can be formal or informal. In some deaneries it is strictly marked, as part of the interview process, whilst in others it is just a chat to ensure that you have matched the required entry criteria. In formal portfolio stations, you may be asked to summarise your experience in 30 seconds, 2 minutes or 5 minutes, to talk about yourself or go through your CV.

The interviewers may also pick on specific areas of your training, asking you to describe in more detail what you did. They may use this opportunity to verify your achievements, i.e. courses, publications or research – bring evidence to support the claims made in your application form.

Motivation, interpersonal skills and NHS issues station
This station deals with your reasons for choosing a specialty or this particular deanery, as well as your communication, team playing and leadership skills. Questions may be general or may ask for specific examples. You may also be asked questions on NHS hot topics relevant to the specialty for which you are being interviewed. In some interviews, NHS issues are addressed at the academic station.

Academic station
The academic station is designed to test your understanding and experience of teaching, research and audit. Questions can be:

- Factual (e.g. "Describe your experience of the audit process", "How do you critically appraise a paper?")

- Reflective (e.g. "What did you gain from your research experience?")

- Probing (e.g. "Do you think that all trainees should do research?").

You may also be asked to critically appraise a paper for which you will have been given anything between 20 and 45 minutes to prepare. Alternatively, you may be asked to discuss a paper you have read recently (make sure you have one you are able to summarise).

If you have undertaken your own research, be prepared to discuss the details and everyday relevance of your publications and thesis.

Clinical governance station

Questions usually revolve around one or more of the following topics:

- Your own understanding of clinical governance and how it affects your practice (e.g. "What do you understand by the term clinical governance?", "How does clinical governance impact on your daily practice?")

- Evidence-based medicine and guidelines (e.g. "What is evidence-based medicine?", "Tell us about a recent paper that you have read", "Tell us about a recent guideline published for this specialty")

- Risk management (e.g. "Tell us about a recent mistake that you have made", "What happens to critical incident forms once you have submitted them?")

- Audit, teaching, research if not already addressed in a separate academic section.

Dilemmas/difficult scenarios station

This station is designed to test your ability to handle difficult problems and dilemmas in the workplace. Questions can take different forms and past interviews have included the following:

- Dealing with two or more important matters at the same time (common in medical interviews, e.g. "you are dealing with an emergency on the ward and you are then called to review another patient urgently on a different ward. How do you prioritise and handle the situation?")

- Dealing with a task for which you are not fully qualified (common in surgical interviews, e.g. "You are in the middle of a surgical procedure and a complication develops. You need to do another procedure, which you have only observed once. What do you do?")

- Dealing with a lack of integrity (for all specialties, e.g. "Your consultant turns up drunk on the ward one morning. What do you do?")

Different specialties and deaneries may structure the stations differently. For example, in 2012, some specialties had only one formal station but it dealt with questions relating to motivation, skills and experience, teamwork, audit and integrity. In many medical specialties, academic and clinical governance questions are often grouped together in one station. The actual structure of the interview matters little. You need to prepare for every type of question regardless of the order in which they are asked.

1.2 Practical interview stations

Practical stations require a much more physical or hands-on involvement from the candidate. In the past they were fairly common in Obstetrics & Gynaecology, Psychiatry and Paediatrics, but nowadays they can be found in almost every specialty.

Communication station
This is more commonly referred to as "role play" or "simulated patient consultation". You are given a small amount of time (5 to 10 minutes) to read a brief, followed by a 10-minute consultation with a patient. The patient is normally played by an actor, though in some cases it has been known to be played by one of the interviewers.

Communication stations deal very specifically with your approach to the patient and the problem rather than your clinical skills, which account only for a small portion of the mark. We address communication stations in Chapter 15.

Presentation station
This station consists of a short presentation (5-10 minutes), often followed in some cases by a question and answer session (also usually 5-10 minutes). In some cases, the topic is given to the candidate on the day (candidates would typically have 45 minutes to prepare); in other cases candidates are given the topic a few days in advance.

Past ST presentation topics have included:

- Generic ("Why would you make a good specialist?")
- Political ("How are current changes affecting the specialty?")
- Personal ("What interests you outside of medicine?").

Chapter 16 details how to handle the presentation station.

Group discussions
Candidates are placed in groups of three or four and are given a topic that they need to debate as a group for usually 20 minutes. There are different types of group discussions, including:

- Simple group discussion around a topic such as a hot topic, how to organise a specific event, etc. In some cases, the discussion can revolve around a document that candidates will have been asked to read before the assessment (e.g. a letter of complaint, a fact sheet relating to a new drug, or even an academic paper)

- Role-based group discussion, where each candidate is playing a different role (e.g. SHO, nurse, manager, patient representative) and must argue their case in relation to a common problem.

We deal with group discussions in Chapter 17.

OSCE (Objective Structured Clinical Examination) station

This assesses your clinical skills (if not already assessed in a separate scenario station). In such a station, you may be asked to examine a patient, take a history or demonstrate a procedure. You may also be asked about the management of specific clinical situations.

Recent examples have included:

- Orthopaedics: naming specific bones handed out at the interview
- Surgery: suturing orange peel or tomato skin
- Anaesthetics: intubating a dummy.

In view of the wide range of specialities, possible clinical scenarios and the practical nature of this station, it would be impossible to deal with this station in a book on interview skills. If you are competent to an appropriate level in your job and can think laterally then you should have no problem in demonstrating your skills in a viva situation and in answering any clinical questions thrown at you. If you have any doubts about your own clinical skills, you may wish to revise using appropriate clinical books and handbooks.

2 Selection criteria

Medical interviews are organised in a "structured" format. Essentially, this means that interviewers are not simply having a general discussion with you (this would be the "unstructured" format that characterised some of the old-style medical interviews), but that they have set out a range of questions designed to test specific skills and competencies. Through the complexity of the interview process, the interviewers will really be assessing three key areas:

- ***Are you competent enough to do the job?*** I.e. do you have the right skills and experience
- ***Do you have the right attitude?*** I.e. do you have the enthusiasm, motivation and drive to be successful in that specialty?
- ***Will you fit in?*** I.e. do you have a personality that will help you get on well both with patients and colleagues in that specialty?

By the time you get to the interview, some of these areas will already have been partially tested through the application form or your CV. The purpose of the form and CV is to act as a first point of selection by looking at the defined essential and desirable criteria. These criteria are detailed in the Person Specifications on the MMC website and are scored according to the scheme in the application pack – this decides the shortlist of candidates for interview.

The appointment committee will use the interview process to determine whether you have the right approach towards your work and a suitable personality. To excel at your interview, you will need to understand the criteria that will be tested so that you can tailor your answers accordingly and ensure that you hit the mark every time.

To gain that understanding, you will need to read two important documents which set out the behaviours and competencies that interviewers will be looking for:

- The National Person Specification of the post for which you are applying.[2]
- The GMC's *Good Medical Practice* (2013).[3]

We discuss both documents over the next few pages and demonstrate their importance throughout the book.

---

[2] www.mmc.nhs.uk

[3] http://www.gmc-uk.org/guidance/good_medical_practice.asp

2.1 National Person Specification

The skills and competencies tested throughout the interview process are set out in a document called the "National Person Specification". Each specialty has its own National Person Specification for each grade. They are made available to candidates with the application form on the MMC website[4] and on individual deanery websites.[5]

The most important part of the National Person Specification for your interview is the section called "Selection Criteria", which summarises the criteria used by the interviewers at the interview. Criteria may vary slightly from grade to grade and from specialty to specialty to reflect the differences in the nature of the work and type of client contact.

I have summarised below those most commonly found and how they may be tested at your interview. For a fully accurate picture, you should read in detail the National Person Specification relevant to the job for which you are applying.

CLINICAL SKILLS

Clinical knowledge & expertise
- Appropriate knowledge base and ability to apply sound clinical judgement to problems
- Able to prioritise clinical need
- Works to maximise safety and minimise risk

Personal attributes
- Shows aptitude for practical skills, e.g. manual dexterity and hand-eye coordination

At the interview, this may be tested by asking you:

- to describe a difficult case that you have managed
- to describe a situation where you had to prioritise clinical needs
- to explain how you would resolve a specific clinical situation
- to prioritise a number of events (e.g. multiple emergencies)
- to analyse test results or images and to describe the next step in the management process
- to demonstrate a given practical skill (e.g. suturing, intubation)
- to demonstrate your understanding of risk management.

---

[4] www.mmc.nhs.uk
[5] see chapter 19

ACADEMIC / RESEARCH SKILLS

Research and audit
- Demonstrates an understanding of the principles and/or importance of research and audit
- Demonstrates an understanding of evidence-based practice
- Evidence of active participation in audit
- Evidence of relevant academic and research achievements

Teaching
- Evidence of interest and experience in teaching

At the interview, this may be tested by asking you:

- to discuss the importance of your research and audit experience
- to explain the difference between audit and research
- to demonstrate your understanding of the audit cycle
- to discuss the usefulness of audit in clinical practice
- to debate the role of research in medical training
- to summarise and analyse a paper that you have read recently
- to explain the principles underlying evidence-based medicine
- to explain research governance or statistical concepts
- to summarise the extent of your teaching experience
- to debate the efficacy of various teaching methods.

JUDGEMENT UNDER / COPING WITH PRESSURE

- Capacity to operate effectively under pressure and remain objective in highly emotive/pressurised situations
- Awareness of own limitations and when to ask for help
- Demonstrates initiative and resilience to cope with changing circumstances

At the interview, this may be tested by asking you:

- to discuss how you handle stress
- to provide an example of a situation where you were stressed
- to explain how you would handle a given stressful scenario
- to give an example of a mistake that you have made
- to talk about a recent situation where you had to ask for senior help or where you felt out of your depth
- to describe a situation where you had to make decisions in a changing environment
- to talk about your weaknesses
- to discuss how you deal with criticism.

COMMUNICATION SKILLS, EMPATHY & SENSITIVITY

Communication skills
- Capacity to communicate effectively and sensitively with others, and ability to discuss treatment options with patients in a way they can understand
- Capacity to adapt language as appropriate to the situation
- Ability to build rapport, listen, influence and negotiate

Empathy & *sensitivity*
- Capacity to take in others' perspectives and treat others with understanding. Sees patients as people

At the interview, communication skills may be tested in different ways. First, the interviewers will be testing your communication skills throughout the interview by assessing how you relate to them, the manner in which you present your answers and how you structure arguments. They will also pick up on non-verbal communication such as your body language, the appropriateness of your tone of voice and the confidence that you exhibit when delivering your answers.

In some specialties, your communication skills, empathy and sensitivity may also be tested through role play (e.g. asking you to explain the management of a condition, to break bad news or to reassure someone) or through a presentation (which will be testing your general communication and teaching skills more than your empathic and sensitive nature).

Finally, you may also be asked direct questions on communication, for example:

- to explain a complex issue in lay terms (e.g. in Ophthalmology, some were asked to explain in lay terms what glaucoma was)
- to describe or rate your communication skills
- to give an example of a situation where your communication skills made a difference to the care of a patient
- to give an example of a situation where you had to deal with a conflict, a difficult colleague/ patient or a vulnerable patient
- to describe how you would handle a situation where one of your colleagues is underperforming.

PROBLEM SOLVING & DECISION MAKING

- Capacity to use logic and lateral thinking to solve problems and make decisions
- Ability to think beyond the obvious, with a flexible mind
- Capacity to bring a range of approaches to problem solving
- Effective judgement and decision-making skills

At an interview, this may be tested by asking you:

- to provide an example of a difficult case that you managed
- to discuss a situation where you had to make a difficult decision (e.g. without senior support)
- to give an example of a situation where you showed initiative
- to describe how you would deal with a difficult given clinical situation.

Problem-solving skills are often tested through clinical questions. In some cases, they may also be tested by discussing difficult scenarios or professional dilemmas.

MANAGING OTHERS, LEADERSHIP & TEAM PLAYING

- Capacity to work effectively in a multidisciplinary team and demonstrate leadership when appropriate
- Capacity to establish good working relations with others
- Ability to supervise junior medical staff

At an interview, this may be tested by asking you:

- to explain what makes you a good team player or team leader
- to provide examples where you have played an important role in a team or where you have shown good leadership
- to detail your experience of working in teams
- to explain what makes a good team and to discuss the advantages and disadvantages of working in teams
- to provide an example of a situation where you had to deal with a difficult situation at work
- to detail your experience of managing others
- to discuss the difference between management and leadership
- to discuss how you delegate and/or to provide examples of delegation and management.

17

ORGANISATION & PLANNING

- Capacity to manage/prioritise time and information effectively
- Capacity to manage time and prioritise workload, to balance urgent and important demands, and to follow instructions
- Capacity to organise ward rounds
- Understands importance and impact of information systems
- Relevant IT skills

At an interview, this may be tested by asking you:

- to explain how you manage your workload or your time
- to provide an example of a situation where you had to prioritise
- to prioritise a list of five or six emergencies or other tasks
- to explain how you would organise a ward round, a theatre list or a training session
- to detail your IT experience and explain its relevance.

VIGILANCE & SITUATIONAL AWARENESS

- Capacity to monitor developing situations and anticipate issues
- Capacity to be alert to dangers or problems, particularly in relation to clinical governance
- Demonstrates awareness of developing situations

At an interview, this may be tested by asking you:

- to provide an example where you showed initiative
- to provide an example of a time when you had to remain vigilant
- to describe a situation when you resolved an unsafe situation
- to explain how you ensure that you remain fully aware of what is happening in complex clinical situations
- to discuss how you would handle a given clinical scenario (e.g. ALS).

2.2 GMC guidance

The GMC's *Good Medical Practice* (2013)

This guidance document sets out the responsibilities of all doctors towards society, their patients and their colleagues. It can be found on the GMC's website (www.gmc-uk.org) and I encourage you to read it before you undertake any preparation as it will crystallise a number of important concepts in your mind.

When doctors talk about *Good Medical Practice* (2013), they often limit their thoughts to the "duties of a doctor", as reproduced in Table 1 on the next page. The "duties of a doctor" are only one part of *Good Medical Practice* (2013) and are essentially a high-level summary of some of the important concepts. *Good Medical Practice* (2013) in fact contains much more than that and attempts to flesh out some of the concepts described in the duties of a doctor.

It is crucial that you spend 30 minutes reading *Good Medical Practice* (2013) attentively on the GMC's website or in the booklet that you should have received from the GMC since, at the interview, you will be expected to demonstrate your understanding of its principles, be it through the provision of examples based on your personal experience, by answering theoretical questions or by discussing difficult scenarios. We will see throughout this book how we can make full use of all this information to transform it into pragmatic, well-structured, well-argued, spontaneous and personal answers.

Other useful guidance

There are, of course, many guidance documents that you will need to be aware of in the course of your career. However, in preparation for your interview, you may want to give priority to the following:

- *Raising and acting on concerns about patient safety* (2012)[6]
- *Confidentiality* (2009)[7]
- *Consent: patients and doctors making decisions together* (2008)[8]

If you are applying for paediatrics or are generally likely to work with children, you may also want to read *0-18 years: guidance for all doctors.*[9]

---

[6] www.gmc-uk.org/guidance/ethical_guidance/raising_concerns.asp
[7] www.gmc-uk.org/guidance/ethical_guidance/confidentiality.asp
[8] www.gmc-uk.org/guidance/ethical_guidance/consent_guidance_index.asp
[9] www.gmc-uk.org/guidance/ethical_guidance/children_guidance_index.asp

Table 1 – Duties of a doctor registered with the General Medical Council

Patients must be able to trust doctors with their lives and health. To justify that trust, you must show respect for human life and make sure your practice meets the standards expected of you in four domains:

Knowledge, skills and performance
- Make the care of your patient your first concern
- Provide a good standard of practice and care
  - Keep your professional knowledge and skills up to date
  - Recognise and work within the limits of your competence

Safety and quality
- Take prompt action if you think that patient safety, dignity or comfort is being compromised
- Protect and promote the health of patients and the public

Communication, partnership and teamwork
- Treat patients as individuals and respect their dignity
  - Treat patients politely and considerately
  - Respect patients' right to confidentiality
- Work in partnership with patients
  - Listen to, and respond to, their concerns and preferences
  - Give patients the information they want or need in a way they can understand
  - Respect patients' right to reach decisions with you about their treatment and care
  - Support patients in caring for themselves to improve and maintain their health
- Work with colleagues in the ways that best serve patients' interests.

Maintaining trust
- Be honest and open and act with integrity
- Never discriminate unfairly against patients or colleagues
- Never abuse your patients' trust in you or the public's trust in the profession

You are personally accountable for your professional practice and must always be prepared to justify your decisions and actions.

Source: www.gmc-uk.org

FORMAL INTERVIEW STATIONS

3   Marking scheme

ST interviews are structured. This means that each question has a specific purpose: to test one or more given skills or competencies. Your answer is then assessed against a range of criteria and marked. This makes it possible to compare candidates in a systematic and objective manner. In essence the rationale behind this design is to make the process fairer; it avoids interviewers drifting down a line of personal interest or grilling candidates unfairly. However, as we will see, there is still room for subjectivity on the part of the interviewer.

The use of a structured marking scheme and the attempt to make interviews more even-handed has led some candidates to assume that there is a "right" answer to questions. That is usually not the case. Interviewers are viewing you as potential long-term colleagues. It is important that you are safe and that you have a good understanding of basic information. To score highly in an interview you will need to be capable of intelligent conversation around issues. This is not possible without the ability to develop and discuss your own opinions and use relevant examples.

Positive and negative indicators

For each question, the interviewers are given a list of positive and negative indicators. Positive indicators are behaviours that one would expect from a suitable candidate. Negative indicators are behaviours that would be cause for concern. For example, if the question is "One of your colleagues is underperforming; what do you do?", the indicators would be along the following lines:

Positive indicators	Negative indicators
<ul><li>Considers impact on patient safety</li><li>Considers the impact on the team and the colleague</li><li>Remains open-minded. Does not judge or jump to conclusions</li><li>Involves appropriate support from/reports appropriately to senior colleagues</li><li>Adopts a supportive and constructive approach</li></ul>	<ul><li>Does not consider impact on patient safety or on the team</li><li>Compromises patient safety</li><li>Handles the problem alone</li><li>Focuses on reporting without measuring the implications on the colleague</li><li>Does not involve appropriate team members</li><li>Judgemental and unsupportive</li></ul>

Similarly, for the question "Describe an example of a time when you had to deal with pressure", positive and negative indicators may be as follows:

Positive indicators	Negative indicators
<ul><li>Demonstrates a positive approach towards the problem</li><li>Considers the wider needs of the situation</li><li>Recognises own limitations</li><li>Is able to compromise</li><li>Is willing to seek help when necessary</li><li>Uses effective strategies to deal with pressure/stress</li></ul>	<ul><li>Perceives challenges as problems</li><li>Attempts unsuccessfully to deal with situation alone</li><li>Uses inappropriate strategies to deal with pressure/stress</li></ul>

If the interviewers feel that there are areas that you have failed to address, they may help you along by probing appropriately.

For example, in answering the question above "Describe an example of a time when you had to deal with pressure", if you focused on how you dealt with the practical/clinical angle of the problem but you forgot to discuss how you managed your stress during and after the event, the interviewers may prompt you with a further question such as "What did you find particularly stressful at the time and how did you handle it?" This would give you an opportunity to present a full picture of your behaviour.

Positive and negative indicators can be imposed centrally (in which case all applicants to the same specialty are judged according to the same indicators, wherever they apply). However, in some cases, each local panel is required to come up with its own positive indicators, which can make the process inconsistent across deaneries.

Marking schedule

Based on the above positive and negative indicators, the interviewers will mark the candidate's performance on a scale of 0 to 4. The marking schedule that is most often used is as follows:

0	No evidence	No evidence reported.
1	Poor	Little evidence of positive indicators. Mostly negative indicators, many decisive

2	Areas for concern	Limited number of positive indicators. Many negative indicators, one or more decisive
3	Satisfactory	Satisfactory display of positive indicators. Some negative indicators but none decisive
4	Good to Excellent	Strong display of positive indicators. Few negative indicators, all minor

This schedule clearly sets a number of criteria in relation to positive and negative indicators. Note that the schedule introduces the concept of "decisive negative indicators". Decisive negative indicators are those which carry a stronger weight than normal because they relate to fundamental problems.

For example, taking an approach that is unsafe for patients would count as a decisive negative indicator. Failing to report a colleague who is endangering patients would also count as a decisive negative factor. In some marking schedules, matching a decisive negative indicator could score you an automatic 0 out of 4. In some interviews, scoring a zero with a decisive negative indicator may trigger an automatic failure of a station or, possibly, the whole interview.

Throughout this book, I will discuss the positive and negative indicators for a wide range of questions. This will give you a good insight into what is expected of you; it will also teach you to work out those indicators by yourself when faced with a question that you did not prepare for or expect.

4 Key interview techniques

Interviews are all about conveying information in a convincing and confident manner. They are therefore, primarily, a communication exercise. It is important that you understand and respect some key principles, which will enable you to present meaningful and confident answers.

Keep your answers between 1½ and 2 minutes

No one can listen to a speaker for more than 2 minutes unless that speaker is absolutely fascinating or has some visual aids to help retain concentration. There is therefore no point in giving answers that are much longer as you run the risk of boring your interviewers.

The only exceptions are open-ended questions, which involve presenting a lot of information (e.g. "Tell us about yourself", "Take us through your CV", "Tell us about your research experience" if you have a lot of it). These may take slightly longer, but you should avoid answers longer than 3 minutes – if you can.

In some (rare) cases, the length of your answers may be strictly dictated by the interviewers. In some specialties, the interview stations last exactly 10 minutes and involve five questions. Allowing for the time taken to ask a question and for interviewers to mark your answers, this leaves about 1½ minutes in which to give an answer. In such cases, the time restriction is usually clearly advertised at the beginning of the process. Make sure that you read carefully any information sent to you prior to the interview.

Make sure also that you consult the appropriate Royal College and deanery websites (see chapter 19) as some deaneries and colleges publish crucial information, including the marking scheme, both for the application and the interview.

Avoid long introductions – answer the question directly

In my experience of interviewing and coaching candidates for interviews, I am often struck by how few people actually answer questions directly. During an interview, it is crucial that you get to the point quickly, address the core of the question and avoid lengthy introductions serving no purpose other than to buy you time.

For example, a typical candidate would start answering a question such as "Tell me about your experience of clinical governance" with the following words "Clinical governance is a framework whereby all organisations …", i.e. by the most common definition. In fact, this does not answer the question. The question is asking for your experience, not a definition or your understanding of governance.

The answer to this question should really start with something along the lines of: "Clinical governance is something that I am involved with on a daily basis. For example, etc…" It is a golden opportunity to showcase how you use tools such as audit, teaching and risk management in your day-to-day practice; do not waste it by reciting a definition – anyone can do this and many will.

Similarly, whenever I have asked someone "How would you describe your communication skills?", the answer has inevitably been: "Communication skills are important in my job because in my specialty we need to communicate every day with a wide range of people, and without communication we cannot be successful. In my day-to-day work I communicate with senior colleagues, junior doctors, nurses, GPs, doctors from other specialties, etc…" Again, this does not answer the question at all.

The candidate is being asked to describe their own communication skills, and not to discuss the importance of communication and the job titles of those to whom they talk. This is not to say that it is totally irrelevant; indeed, such information may have a place in the final answer, but using it at length right at the start of the answer will irritate the interviewers. Instead, the candidate should talk about how good they think they are, the aspects of communication they are particularly good at, and the feedback they have received.

The answer should start much more directly, with something like: "I feel that I have good communication skills and the feedback that I have received both from my patients and my colleagues has been extremely positive." This would then be followed by three or four points setting out the candidate's strengths in communication.

As a rule it is sensible to avoid using abbreviations – even familiar ones. From a communication point of view they can sound sloppy and lazy. You may also confuse members of your panel – especially if there are lay members present.

Structure your answers in three or four points

A problem that plagues candidates is the lack of structure in their answers. This makes it difficult for the interviewers to identify easily what the candidate is getting at. The human brain finds it difficult to remember more than three or four ideas at a time; so there is no point in giving your interviewers ten different ideas in the same answer. You will struggle to recall them and it will only confuse your panel. Stick to three or four points maximum. If you feel you need more than four points to say what you want to say, then see if you can structure your answer in a different manner.

For example, the answer to "Tell us about your teaching experience" can be structured as follows:

- Who you have taught, what you taught them and how often
- Which teaching methods you have experience of
- Teaching courses you have attended
- Feedback you have received.

The answer to "Tell us about a mistake that you have made" can be structured along these lines:

- Description of the scenario and the mistake made
- How you dealt with the mistake at the time
- What you learnt from the incident/how it changed your practice
- How you made sure others learnt too (including critical incident reporting)

The answer to "What are your main strengths?" can be structured using three personality traits, which are sufficiently different to justify being placed in different sections. For example:

- Dynamic and proactive
- Approachable and supportive
- Self-starter and constantly willing to learn and develop.

Each of the points can then be developed individually. The clear and succinct structure will leave no doubt as to where you are going with your answer. Not only will a strong structure enable the interviewers to understand what you are saying without putting in too much effort, it will also make you sound much more direct, engaging and confident.

Expand on each point and illustrate with examples

It is all too easy to quote a few buzzwords and to think that they will be sufficient to tick all the right boxes. For example, many candidates answer the question "What makes you a good doctor?" with the following one-liner: "I am a good doctor because I am hardworking, motivated, dedicated, focused, a good communicator, a good team player, I learn from experience and constantly seek to develop new skills". None of these words are wrong and indeed, strictly speaking, this sentence answers the question asked. However, a succession of buzzwords can make the answer sound clichéd and impersonal. In fact, every candidate could give the same answer regardless of their grade and specialty.

Making broad statements makes you sound vague (and possibly arrogant); it also makes it difficult for interviewers to positively differentiate you from other candidates. It is therefore crucial to back up any claims you make with examples drawn from personal experience; this will leave no doubt in anyone's mind about your abilities.

For example, "I learn from experience and constantly seek to develop new skills" is an easy statement to make. Once you have made this statement, you could recall briefly one or two examples where this happened, as follows:

"From the very beginning of my training, I have taken every opportunity to learn from and build on my experience. For example, recently I had trouble getting a patient to agree to a procedure and with the help of my registrar I learnt to take a different communication approach which I have now incorporated into my practice.

Whenever I encounter clinical situations with which I am less comfortable than others, I take the time to read up on it and in fact often volunteer to run teaching sessions on those difficult topics. Recently I have identified that a couple of local guidelines were no longer appropriate and I volunteered to update them.

During that process, I learnt a lot not only about how to conduct literature reviews, but also how to communicate with colleagues, as some members of the team showed a reluctance to change their established practices.

Following on from that, I took it upon myself to attend a Trust-run management course and I have since taken on other projects such as <xxx>."

Bringing examples into your answers makes you sound more mature and practical; it also enables you to discuss other skills. For example, the answer above brings in management and leadership and shows that you are in control.

Signpost each point clearly – make your points clear

Signposting means stating clearly the new concept or idea that you are addressing. Many candidates have answers that are well structured and contain a lot of interesting information backed up with good examples; however, in spite of this, it can still be difficult to extract the message or idea they are trying to communicate from their answer. This section aims to help you to clarify your message. Once you have a structure in mind, make sure your key messages are announced clearly within each section of your answer. These may be introduced in a number of ways, as illustrated below.

- ***Signposting at the start***
  Signposting is more easily done at the start of each section. For example, an answer to the question "Why do you want to train in surgery?" could consist of three sections signposted as follows:

Introduction	"There are many reasons why I am keen to train as a surgeon.
Signpost & Expand	First, I draw a lot of personal satisfaction from being able to make an immediate difference to my patients. <Then explain why and how, bring examples>
Signpost & Expand	As well as this, I also have a strong interest in research and I feel that surgery is an excellent specialty in which to pursue that interest. <Then expand explaining what the interest consists of and how this relates to a career in surgery>
Signpost & Expand	Finally, I really enjoy working under pressure and in close cooperation with other colleagues." <Then expand on how this is important in surgery and what you enjoy about it>

In this example, each section starts with a clear message, which is what the candidate wants the interviewers to remember about him/her.

- ***Signposting at the end***
  Signposting can also be done at the end of each section of an answer. In this case, the candidate would typically start the section with a description of his experience and would then conclude by explaining how this is relevant to the question asked. For example, for the question "Why do you want to train in surgery", instead of stating up front that he/she has a strong interest in research, the candidate could phrase the answer as follows:

| Context/Experience | "During my attachment in Orthopaedics I had an opportunity to become involved in two research projects, one which was on <xxx> and another one on <yyy>. Through my involvement in these projects, I gained a good insight into different research methodologies and the importance of research overall, and I discovered that I felt very much at ease both in the clinical and the academic setting. |

Signpost/Message	I feel that surgery is a field that will provide an ideal opportunity to apply both my clinical and academic skills to patient care."

This would then be followed by two more sections dealing with other reasons for choosing surgery as a career. In this example, the message is clearly stated in the last sentence, leaving the interviewers with no ambiguity as to what the candidate is trying to say.

- *Vary the signposting*
Beginning all sections of all answers with a signpost is likely to make you sound slightly "military" or overly systematic. Signposting all sections at the end may give the feeling that you are constantly trying to build suspense and drama in your answers.

If you can, i.e. if you feel confident enough to do so, try to vary the way in which you signpost so that some of your answers have points that are signposted at the start and others at the end. This will give a more balanced picture and will be easier on the ear of your panel.

However, if you do not feel able to vary your answers in this way, stick to signposting at the start. It is the easier of the two to master. Once you feel more comfortable, you can start experimenting and softening your delivery by mixing the two styles.

Use power words and active verbs

Selling yourself is not just about stating your message clearly and describing your experience. It is also about sounding confident, mature and, generally speaking, in control. It is a common mistake for candidates to understate their experience. In order to appear more confident, you will need to adopt a vocabulary which may be slightly different to that which you are accustomed to on a day-to-day basis, and which will sell you in an active and enthusiastic manner.

There is no need to learn a whole list of words in order to achieve this. When you are preparing your answers to some of the more common questions, particularly those based on your personal experience, you should question whether your answers sound energetic and enthusiastic enough. If they don't, this could be a problem with the structure or a lack of personalisation in your answer; but it could also be due to the lack of power words and active verbs.

Example

Consider this sentence: "After a few attempts, I was able to reach a compromise with my colleagues."

On the surface, it sounds like a good thing to say. However, "After a few attempts" and "I was able to" sound weak. They make it sound as if the candidate didn't try that hard or is not particularly proud of their achievement.

The sentence could have a much stronger impact if it were reworded as follows: "Following several discussions where I encouraged my colleagues to review their position, I was successful in helping the team reach a compromise."

In this revised sentence, the words "encouraged" and "successful" present a much more proactive candidate and make a big difference in the manner in which the answer is being received by the listener.

Try to reconsider your answers and experiment with inserting words from the comprehensive list of over 500 power words in section 18. Your answers will become more punchy and interesting.

Talk about yourself, rather than everyone else

Candidates who feel uncomfortable at interviews usually compensate by talking about everything else but themselves. They talk repeatedly about "we" and "the team" and, although it does present a good team-playing attitude, it fails to demonstrate their personal skills and competencies.

In your interview, it is perfectly acceptable to introduce some collective actions and make statements such as "As a team, we were charged with conducting an audit on waiting times in A&E". This sentence should only serve as an introduction to the rest of the answer, which then remains focused on you and no one else with the use of "I", "My responsibilities", "My aim", etc.

Bring objectivity into your answers

If you feel awkward talking about yourself or don't want to appear boastful, a good way to overcome this problem is to bring objectivity into your answers. This can be achieved by:

- Illustrating your answers with personal examples and
- Mentioning feedback that you have received, either informally or through 360-degree appraisal.

Instead of "I feel that I am an excellent listener", you may feel more comfortable saying "My patients and colleagues have often commented on the fact that I am a very good listener."

31

Avoid making vague statements

Keep to statements that provide definite, factual information. Avoid vague statements such as "I went into surgery because I like it" unless you can back up your statement. What really matters is why you find it interesting or why you like it. Use facts to substantiate your general statements. Use the 5 "W" questions (what, who, where, when, why) and the "H" question (how) to gain knowledge about yourself and add content.

Avoid unnecessary detail

Avoid excessive detail when giving examples unless you have been asked for specifics. If you provide too much intricate detail, your answer will be very long and wordy. Most importantly, you will distract from your key message by concentrating on one issue whilst the question may be much broader.

Remain positive

Whether I coach people who are applying for CT, ST, Consultant, Clinical or Medical Director posts, or even higher up, candidates incriminate themselves by delivering answers with a negative undertone right from the start. I have lost count of the number of people who start their answers to the question "What is your research experience?" by saying "Well, I haven't done much research"; or those who describe their communication skills as "above average", i.e. nothing special. To make an impact, you must sell what you have rather than what you don't have. If you don't show that you believe in yourself then no one else will.

5 Key interview structures and frameworks

In order to produce structured and meaningful answers, you will need to learn to use a number of structures and frameworks that will make your life easier. Once you have mastered these, you will be able to apply them endlessly across a wide range of questions. Not only will this give you a sense of direction, it will also provide you with reassurance as you deliver your answers. You will feel more in control because you will know that there are sound principles that you can apply, regardless of what the question is.

In this section, I introduce three fundamental structures:

- **CAMP**: for background and motivation questions

- **STAR**: for skills-based questions asking for specific examples

- **SPIES**: to answer questions on difficult colleagues or conflicts.

Make sure that you do not simply memorise these techniques but that you learn to use them intelligently – the next level beyond the use of acronyms to simply remember, for example, the cranial nerves or branches of the internal iliac artery. At the interview, you are likely to feel nervous and to blank out if you simply try to recall information. The key to success is to allow sufficient time to prepare so that these structures become second nature and you do not have so much thinking and information-recalling to do on the spot.

Throughout the book, I will apply these key generic structures and will also develop other structures that are more specific to individual questions. More importantly, I will show you how to think about the questions logically and construct answers using your common sense and experience.

5.1 The CAMP structure (for background & motivation questions)

CAMP = Clinical, Academic, Management, Personal

When answering questions such as "Tell me about yourself", "Take me through your CV", "Why do you want to train in this deanery?" (for training posts), or any generic question which draws on the breadth of your experience, CAMP will provide you with a ready-made structure that will enable you to provide a logical and well-developed answer.

For example, when answering the question "How do you see your career developing over the next 10 years?", using the CAMP structure will prompt you for ideas along the following lines:

Clinical   You may want to work in a specific type of hospital (e.g. teaching, DGH, tertiary hospital). You may also want to develop special clinical skills or interests.

Academic   You may have an academic interest and want to develop research interests and skills. You may be keen on teaching and want to get involved in education and training activities. You may even wish to get involved at regional or royal college level, and perhaps undertake a medical education degree.

Management   You may want to gain further experience in areas such as service development, audit, or risk management. Perhaps, even, you are aiming at becoming an educational supervisor or other responsibilities.

Personal   Is there a region where you would like to settle? Perhaps you would like to spend some time abroad to expand your horizons both clinically and socially. Do you have any relevant or interesting hobbies or skills that will make your interviewers want to ask you more?

5.2   The STAR structure (for questions asking for an example)

STAR = Situation, Task, Action, Result/Reflect

The STAR structure is a universally recognised communication technique designed to provide meaningful and complete answers to questions asking for specific examples, such as:

- "Tell us about a situation where you worked under pressure"
- "Describe a situation when you dealt with a difficult patient"
- "Tell us about a time when you played a key role in a team"
- "Describe a situation where you had to ask for senior help"
- "Give an example where your communication skills made a difference to the care of a patient."

Many interviewers will have been trained to use this structure. Even if they have not, they will recognise its value when they see it. The information will be given to them in a structured manner and, as a result, they will become more receptive to the messages you are trying to communicate.

The interviewers will be looking for the following:

Situation	What is the context of the story?
Task	What did you have to achieve?
Action	What did you do? How did you go about achieving it? And why did you do it in that way?
Result/**R**eflect	What happened at the end? Why did you feel you did well? If the example is about a mistake or a difficult situation, what did you learn? How did it change you?

Step 1 – Situation or Task

Describe the situation that you were confronted with or the task that needed to be accomplished. This section is merely setting the scene for the "Action" section so that your panel can understand the story from start to finish. You should therefore aim to make it concise and informative, concentrating solely on what is pertinent to the story and the message you are trying to communicate.

For example, if the question is asking you to describe a situation where you had to deal with a difficult person, explain how you came to meet that person and why they were being difficult. If the question is asking for an example of teamwork, explain the task that you had to undertake as a team and what your role was.

Step 2 – Action

This is the most important section as it is where you will need to demonstrate that you have the skills and personal attributes that the question is testing. Having set the context of your story, you need to explain the action you took, bearing in mind the following:

- Be personal, i.e. talk about you, not other people
- Go into some detail. Do not assume that the interviewers will guess what you mean
- Steer clear of clinical information, unless it is essential for the general comprehension of the story
- Explain not just what you did, but how and why you did it.

What you did and how you did it

Explain the actions that you took to resolve the situation, highlighting clearly your role. In describing your role, keep in mind the purpose of the question and the skills that it is asking you to demonstrate.

For example, a question asking you to provide an example of a situation when you dealt with a difficult patient will involve discussing a number of points, including:

- How you used your communication skills effectively
- How you sought to involve others in helping you deal with the patient
- How you dealt with your frustration.

Why you did it

If you stick to explaining what you did and how you did it, you run the risk of giving an answer that is slightly too basic. In your answer, you must be able to demonstrate that you are taking actions because you understand their purpose and what they will achieve, not simply because you got lucky.

Never lose sight of the fact that the example is only of interest if you demonstrate through your narration how you match the desired criteria.

Consider the following question and (ineffective) answer:

Question:
"Tell me about a time where you dealt with a difficult patient."

Ineffective answer:
"I was called to Accident and Emergency to review a patient who, I'd been told, was aggressive and abusive towards other patients and even towards members of staff. I came down to Accident and Emergency and took the patient to a separate room. We had a 10-minute discussion during which I was able to resolve his problem. The patient left shortly thereafter and decided not to make a complaint."

This example is very superficial. On the positive side it does follow the STAR structure but, although the candidate has described what they did, there is a distinct lack of detail.

More importantly, we do not know why they acted in this way and what they were trying to achieve. This will make it difficult to mark the candidate appropriately. For example, why did they take the patient to a separate room? By highlighting the reasons behind their reaction, the candidate would make a greater impact, as follows:

Reworded partial answer
"...As I arrived in Accident and Emergency, there were two issues that I needed to address. My main priority was to ensure that the staff and patients who had been abused were unharmed so I asked a senior nurse to look after them. Meanwhile, I was also conscious of the need to take the patient away from the emotions of the situation so that we could have a sensible discussion about the issues at stake. I felt that the best way to address this was to take him to a separate room, taking another colleague with me for my own safety..."

By explaining both what you did and the reasons behind your actions, you bring more depth to your answers and will appear a more mature candidate and consequently score much higher.

Step 3 – Result

Explain what happened eventually: how it all ended. You may be surprised by the number of candidates who finish their answers on a cliff-hanger. By not concluding your story, you will leave the interviewers with a strange sensation and, although they are likely to prompt you for an ending and a reflection, it will sound much better if you come to it of your own accord.

Once you have stated the ending of the story, you can then conclude the answer in two different ways:

- By reflecting on the scenario and explaining the significance of the story to your role as a doctor

> **Example of an ending for the question: "Tell me about a time where you dealt with a difficult patient."**
>
> "...After our discussion, the patient decided not to make a complaint and said that he was actually very happy with the attention that he had received. By focusing my attention on the needs of the patient and the safety of the staff, I was able to redress the situation successfully. This example demonstrated how important simple things like listening can be, and how much can go wrong when communication is not properly handled."

- By summarising the key skills you demonstrated during the scenario

> **Example of an ending for the question: "Give us an example of a situation where you showed leadership."**
>
> "...Throughout this scenario, I showed leadership both by ensuring that all junior members of the team knew exactly what they had to do and that they were supported in their role by my availability if there were problems. I also ensured that my seniors were kept fully up to date with key developments and that we not only took care of the patient's needs but also of the relatives' needs for information and support."

5.3 The SPIES structure (for questions on difficult colleagues)

SPIES = Seek info, Patient safety, Initiative, Escalate, Support

Questions asking how you would deal with a difficult colleague come in different shapes and forms. The level of difficulty varies from simple lateness to training-related underperformance and attitude problems, to sheer criminal acts. In these questions, the level of seniority of the colleague in question also varies from a junior doctor to someone more senior, such as a consultant, for example.

Examples of questions frequently asked include:

- "One of your junior colleagues keeps coming in late. What do you do?"
- "What would you do if your consultant came into the ward/theatre drunk one morning?"
- "One of your colleagues keeps turning up 20 minutes late each morning. What do you do?"
- "Your consultant is asking you to do something that you feel is wrong (e.g. modifying notes to cover up a mistake). What do you do?"
- "Your Registrar constantly fails to answer his bleep, leaving you several times in precarious situations. He tells you that his batteries keep going flat. What do you do?"
- "During a break in the mess, you see a bag of cocaine fall out of your Registrar's pocket. How do you handle the situation?"
- "You walk into your consultant's office and see him watching images of child pornography on the hospital computer. What do you do?"

The scenarios are daunting and these questions often strike fear into the heart of candidates – most of us imagine the worst case and the thought of having to remove our drunken boss from the ward. Psychologically, part of the difficulty is to overcome the fear of what would happen to "me" if I blew the whistle. Your interviewers will demand that you understand the broad implications of the scenario not only for patients, but also for the team and for your colleague. They will be testing your ability to address all the relevant issues appropriately. Having the SPIES structure as a basis for your answer allows you to deal with any of the above questions by applying the same principles.

At the interview, you will be expected to demonstrate that you can handle the situation in a responsible and mature manner, ensuring patient safety at all times whilst also resolving the matter sensitively.

To ensure that you cover all angles, you will need to consider the following:

Seek info	Before you can do anything, you need to understand the nature of the problem. In some cases, it will take a fraction of a second (e.g. if a colleague is drunk). In others, it may take longer (e.g. if a colleague does not appear motivated). This may involve discussing the matter with the individual concerned or with other colleagues, if appropriate.
Patient Safety	Once you have assessed the situation, you must make sure that patients are protected. If the person is an immediate threat to patients (e.g. drunk or about to do the wrong operation), then you must remove them from the clinical area or tell them to stop doing whatever they are doing (this could be done by having a quiet word with the individual in question, or in the worst-case scenario calling for help to have them removed).
Initiative	Is there anything that you can do by yourself that will help resolve the problem? In practice, this will only apply to minor issues, where there is no real threat to patient safety.
	If the colleague is drunk, there is little that you can do to help. However, if it is just an issue of a junior colleague being a bit slow, then there are things that you could do to help out in the first instance (e.g. individual coaching or a discussion).
Escalate	If the situation is too serious for you to deal with, then you must involve other colleagues at appropriate levels of seniority. For a problem junior colleague, this could be the Registrar, the education supervisor of the underperforming colleague or another consultant.
	For an underperforming consultant, this would need to be the clinical director. If the situation is not resolved, you may need to escalate further to the medical director, the chief executive or even the GMC. If you don't know what to do, you can seek advice from other organisations (e.g. the BMA, any medical defence organisation, the GMC).
Support	There are reasons for the colleague to behave in this way. As an individual he will need support to deal with the problem. Your team will also need support if it is one person down.

This approach is supported by the following articles from the GMC's guidance documents:

Good Medical Practice (2013) – Article 25:
"You must take prompt action if you think that patient safety, dignity or comfort is or may be seriously compromised.

a. If a patient is not receiving basic care to meet their needs, you must immediately tell someone who is in a position to act straight away.

b. If patients are at risk because of inadequate premises, equipment or other resources, policies or systems, you should put the matter right if that is possible. You must raise your concern in line with our guidance and your workplace policy. You should also make a record of the steps you have taken.

c. If you have concerns that a colleague may not be fit to practise and may be putting patients at risk, you must ask for advice from a colleague, your defence body or us. If you are still concerned, you must report this, in line with our guidance and your workplace policy, and make a record of the steps you have taken."

Raising and acting on concerns about patient safety (2012) – Article 12
"If you have reason to believe that patients are, or may be, at risk of death or serious harm for any reason, you should report your concern to the appropriate person or organisation immediately. Do not delay doing so because you yourself are not in a position to put the matter right."

Raising and acting on concerns about patient safety (2012) – Article 13
"Wherever possible, you should first raise your concern with your manager or an appropriate officer of the organisation you have a contract with or which employs you – such as the consultant in charge of the team, the clinical or medical director or a practice partner. If your concern is about a partner, it may be appropriate to raise it outside the practice – for example, with the medical director or clinical governance lead responsible for your organisation. If you are a doctor in training, it may be appropriate to raise your concerns with a named person in the deanery – for example, the postgraduate dean or director of postgraduate general practice education."

Good Medical Practice (2013) – Article 43:
"You must support colleagues who have problems with their performance or health. But you must put patient safety first at all times."

As we will see throughout this book when we study individual questions dealing with problem doctors or difficult colleagues, a lot of the answers call upon your common sense. The SPIES structure is really there to make sure that you do not forget anything crucial in your answers.

6 Portfolio station

Many ST interviews contain a separate portfolio station where the interviewers will go through the various sections of the candidate's portfolio and ask relevant questions. In some cases portfolio stations are merely a formality but in many others they are actually a formal station with a formal marking schedule. Either way, the importance of this station should not be underestimated.

Even an informal set-up will involve careful checks of your CV – including any publications or achievements you have listed. As well as any documents you are told to bring, take along evidence of your achievements, including copies of papers or posters (an A4 version is fine). If you are writing or have written a thesis, bring along what you have done – if it is complete that looks fantastic; if you have written chunks of it, that shows a mark of intent.

Historically, there have been examples of candidates exaggerating their achievements – part of this station's role is to pick that up. It is not unheard of for panels to perform a literature search on candidates – if you are honest you have nothing to fear but a lie will fail you that interview and may land you in front of the GMC.

The scoring system varies from specialty to specialty, as well as between deaneries. However, it is commonly as follows:

Oral presentation and communication skills (5 marks)

The candidate will be asked to talk about specific aspects of their experience such as a specific job or rotation. Questions may also be broader; in many portfolio questions, candidates are asked to take the interviewers through their CV or to talk about themselves in no more than 2, 3 or 5 minutes depending on the circumstances (see 7.1 and 7.2 for details on how to answer these). Candidates are assessed on their fluency and verbal communication. A lack of structure and coherence, as well as poor eye contact, will usually ensure the lowest mark.

Interaction with the panel (5 marks)

As the panel questions candidates about their experience, they will be assessing the candidate's ability to consider the questions asked and the relevance of the answers provided. An ability to think quickly, provide relevant answers and communicate effectively would lead to a high mark, whilst a lack of coherence and relevance would ensure a low mark.

Quality of competence evidence (5 marks)

The panel will be assessing the evidence presented by the candidate to vouch for his competence (log book, DOPs, mini-CEX, etc.) and will be judging the organisation, layout, presentation, legibility and completeness of the information. A low score would be given for poor evidence or unclear layout.

Quality of CV (5 marks)

As well as the evidence, the panel will be assessing the quality and layout of the candidate's CV. A comprehensive and well-presented CV with fully relevant information will score highly, whilst a disorganised CV with poor evidence will score low.

7 Background & motivation questions

7.1 Take me through your CV

In answering this question, it is tempting to list your experience methodically. However, this is unlikely to result in a very engaging and enthusiastic answer and would certainly take more than the allocated time to deliver your full biography. The following rules will enable you to provide a comprehensive yet concise and personal answer.

Do not literally take them through the CV

I remember once sitting in on an interview where the candidate actually started his answer with: "Well, on the 1st page, you will find my name, address and qualifications; on the 2nd page, the list of past jobs, etc." Needless to say, the panel was not impressed. Instead of boring everyone with a lengthy description of every page, think of the themes that your CV addresses and of the points that you want the interviewers to remember about you.

Do not worry about overlapping with future questions

Many candidates worry that, if they talk about everything at the start of the interview, they will have nothing else to say later on if they are asked a question on research or teaching, for example. In reality, you simply do not know what questions you will be asked later on, so do not deprive your interviewers of important information on that basis. Treat this question as a contents table for the interview, where you will be setting out what you have to offer in a logical and structured manner, without going into excessive detail.

Avoid the chronological approach

Structuring your whole answer around the chronology of your training to date will create an answer which will feel long and in which you will spend much time listing hospital names, dates and specialty names. Going through every single job you have had so far may be okay if you have very few jobs behind you, but if you have more than five or six then it could prove lengthy. The most effective answers tend to be structured around the main themes of a candidate's experience (i.e. their clinical training, why they enjoy the specialty, their research and audit experience, etc.) rather than the chronology of their training.

Apply the CAMP structure (see 5.1)

If your CV is well designed, it will already have been written more or less along the lines of the CAMP structure (i.e. with clinical information at the start; followed by your audit, research, teaching and management experience; finishing with more personal information such as hobbies). There is no reason why the answer to this question should vary widely from the actual structure of your CV. You simply need to convert it into something that is easy to listen to. Here is an example of how you could structure your answer:

Clinical
- Brief chronology of your training (15/20 seconds)
- Description of skills and experience (2 to 4 points)
- How this motivated you for this specialty/post, or why you want to train in this specialty.

Academic
Brief description of your research/teaching involvement, including:
- Papers you have written
- Relevant postgraduate qualifications
- Postgraduate courses you have been on
- Teaching you have done, teaching qualifications or courses
- A summary of your intercalated degree or postgraduate thesis (if you have done one)
- Any grants you have won.

Management
- Brief description of your audit experience
- Overview of your other management experience, including:
  - Rota management
  - Service development or service improvement including conducting audits and implementing changes thereafter
  - Experience of writing or updating guidelines and protocols
  - Sitting on committees, e.g. risk management
  - Acting as representative, e.g. junior doctors committee
  - Handling complaints (for more senior candidates)
  - Organising events, including induction programmes for junior doctors or nurses, departmental or regional teaching programmes, mock exams, conferences, etc.
  - Dealing with underperforming colleagues (for more senior candidates, e.g. ST3)
  - Any other management experience linked to a personal achievement or outside medicine.

Personal

- Overview of your personal strengths/interpersonal skills
- Basic information about your social life (e.g. hobbies).

Example of an effective answer

"My name is John. I am currently training as an FY2 doctor in the East of England deanery. I graduated in 2011 from Cambridge University. I have trained in the Eastern region for both foundation years, during which I have experienced a range of specialties, including Cardiology, Respiratory, Accident and Emergency, Obstetrics and Gynaecology, and General Practice. Out of all of these, I have particularly enjoyed the medical specialties because of the analytical and communication challenges that they offer and this is the reason that I am applying to Core Medical Training.

During medical school and the ensuing two foundation years, I have gained a lot of confidence in history taking and basic procedures such as cannulation, ABG sampling and urethral catheterisation. Through my cardiology attachment, I gained a good knowledge of ECG interpretation. I was able to perform cardiac catheterisation under supervision, I assisted in the placement of pacing wires and I took the opportunity to observe transoesophageal echocardiography. My A&E attachment helped to increase my confidence in dealing with acutely ill patients; it also provided me with excellent training in how to remain calm and organised under pressure, which has proved extremely useful during my on-call work.

As well as developing good clinical skills, I have sought to develop my teaching skills. I have been involved in teaching undergraduates on basic clinical matters and procedures with both bedside or ward teaching and formal lectures. I have also actively sought to mentor groups of medical students who have rotated through the units I have worked in. Teaching is something that interests me greatly, and which I'd be keen to develop further throughout my training and my career.

Over the past few years, I have also played an active role in audit projects. I have completed two audits, one of which led to a change in clinical practice through the introduction of new departmental guidelines for the follow-up of MI patients. On both audits, I was the lead auditor. As well as this, I have played a key role in organising departmental activities, including a weekly departmental teaching session and some mock vivas for medical students in their final year.

From a more personal perspective, my colleagues see me as someone who is reliable and very supportive. Outside of work, I enjoy team sports such as football and cricket, which give me an outlet to de-stress. I also enjoy reading and spending time out with friends."

This answer takes about 2 minutes to deliver at a realistic enthusiastic pace. Slower candidates (and speaking slowly is by no means a disadvantage) could easily deliver an answer of this length in 2½ minutes.

Why this answer works

- It is well structured. You will have recognised that it follows the CAMP structure. The short introduction where the doctor gives his name and his current post is very effective. Obviously, they should already know your name, but the purpose of this sentence is not to provide information. It is designed to build a rapport. They won't know you at all; so it is nice to introduce yourself.

- The candidate does not just list information or make bold statements about having experience. It is easy to make statements such as "I have gained a lot of audit and teaching experience", hoping that interviewers might understand what was meant by it. Instead, the candidate provides concrete examples of achievements.

- The candidate ends his answer with a more personal slant. Note the use of feedback: "my colleagues see me as someone who is reliable and very supportive." With such a sentence, there is an immediate picture of someone who works well in a team, even though they have never actually said "I am a good team player".

- The information has opened up several avenues of interest that the interviewers can then follow with questions. The information is accurate and punchy: just enough of an appetiser for the panel to gain a feeling of confidence about the candidate.

Ending the answer

In this example, the candidate finished with the personal section. His tone of voice should clearly indicate that he has finished the answer. Another possible finish would involve taking out the sentence: "Out of all of these, I have particularly enjoyed the medical specialties because of the analytical and communication challenges that they offer and this is the reason that I am applying to Core Medical Training" from the first paragraph, and to position it instead in the last paragraph in a slightly modified format:

> "Out of all my attachments and training opportunities so far, I have enjoyed the medical specialties most because of the analytical and communication challenges that they offer; and this is the reason that I am applying to Core Medical Training."

7.2 Tell me about yourself

This question puzzles many candidates, whose first reaction is to ask back "What do you want me to talk about? Do you want to know about my training, my research, my hobbies?"

If you ask the interviewers to narrow the scope of the question, you will lose a valuable opportunity to demonstrate your full potential. You may also give the impression that you are unable to determine what is important and what is less important to the interviewers, which may then raise questions about your ability to prioritise information.

The purpose of the interview is to determine whether you are the right candidate for the post. Focusing an answer on your hobbies or your personality will not enable you to sell yourself fully. You should aim to tick as many boxes as you can and use the vagueness of the question to your advantage by presenting your strengths, skills and achievements.

The good news is that, if you have already prepared "Take me through your CV", there is little further preparation to do. Indeed, these two questions are essentially the same and you can deliver the same answer in exactly the same way.

7.3 Why do you want to train in this specialty?

What the interviewers are looking for

This question is testing your motivation for the post and the interviewers will be looking for the following:

- A range of reasons: some marking schemes take into account the number of reasons listed. To ensure that you maximise your score, you will need to state at least three, preferably four. Any more than four and you run the risk of spreading your answer too thin or repeating yourself. You should also ensure that your reasons are sufficiently different from one another so that you do not sound repetitive and the answer has enough variety to keep the interviewers interested throughout.

- Strong explanations, with a personal slant: simply listing your reasons for choosing the specialty will not be sufficient. You need to explain why these reasons are important to you and how you developed your interest.

- Evidence that demonstrates your interest in the specialty: thinking that a specialty will suit you is not enough. The interviewers will be looking for evidence that you have taken steps to test your interest or to gain experience in that specialty. These posts are precious opportunities and your panel wants to know that you are going to make good use of the opportunity if it is given to you.

- Career focus: your choice of specialty needs to come across as something that you have thought about and fits within a career plan. The interviewers will not be keen on recruiting someone who wants to join the specialty because "it sounds quite interesting" or because they could not get into anything else.

- Enthusiasm: it is not a competition about who will have the best reason or the most reasons; it is about recruiting those who believe in their future in the specialty. This can only be achieved by talking, in some detail, about what you enjoy. Some of the enthusiasm will be conveyed through your description of your experience to date; but most of it will come from your tone of voice and the enthusiastic manner with which you deliver your answer.

Defining your reasons for training in the specialty

Statements such as "I want to train in this specialty because I find it interesting, stimulating, fascinating, enriching, etc." are common and not particularly informative. Adjectives such as "interesting" and "fascinating" may sound good on the surface, but they are meaningless unless you explain why you find the specialty interesting or fascinating. Use such words sparingly, particularly as most of your competitors will overuse them and the interviewers will be bored of hearing them time after time.

Your answer should be structured around three or four clear reasons. These reasons will of course depend on your personal circumstances and the specialty. For this question, you can also use the CAMP structure (see 5.1) as a useful tool to ensure that you cover all angles. Here are a few examples that you can use as a starting point:

Clinical reasons
- The technological aspect (e.g. surgery, radiology, pathology)
- The variety of work that the specialty offers, for example:
    - You deal with different specialties (e.g. Paediatrics)
    - Good mix of medicine and surgery (e.g. Ophthalmology, Obstetrics & Gynaecology)
    - A mix of ward work and clinics (most medical specialties)
    - A mix of chronic and acute patients
    - Involves prevention as well as treatment
    - Mix of interventional and other activities (e.g. Cardiology, Radiology)
    - Opportunity to work in different settings (e.g. community and hospital for Psychiatry, Paediatrics, GUM)
- You get immediate results from your work (e.g. most surgical specialties). Be careful with this reason because surgeons also deal with chronic patients. A better reason may be that you enjoy the combination of the two.
- A strong investigative component, or, on the other hand, there aren't many investigations available so it offers you a challenge.
- The diagnosis is easy to establish, or on the contrary it is challenging.
- The holistic/psychosocial approach (e.g. Psychiatry, Oncology).

Academic reasons (research, teaching)
- Fast advancing specialty, with a real challenge in keeping up to date and constantly learning new skills (e.g. most surgical specialties, Oncology)
- Good opportunities for research
- Good opportunities for teaching
- Great variety in teaching styles (e.g. simulation in Anaesthetics)
- Opportunity to develop a special interest.

Management Reasons (responsibility, working with others)
- Opportunities to get involved rapidly in areas of responsibility where one has greater autonomy (e.g. Psychiatry)
- Strong multidisciplinary focus (e.g. Psychiatry, Paediatrics, Oncology)
- Mix of independent work and teamwork
- Opportunities to develop services and make a real difference to service provision

- Prefer to work in small teams and therefore hold greater responsibilities (e.g. Dermatology, Haematology, Urology)

Personal reasons (personality, soft skills, social)
- Offers a communication challenge (e.g. Paediatrics, Psychiatry)
- The challenge of dealing with difficult patients and sensitive situations (e.g. Paediatrics, Psychiatry, Obstetrics & Gynaecology)
- Your input has a strong influence on patient satisfaction: makes a big difference to the patient's lifestyle and mobility (e.g. Ophthalmology, Orthopaedics) and therefore leads to greater satisfaction
- The buzz of working under pressure (e.g. surgery, emergency medicine)
- Enjoy working in an environment where detail matters (e.g. Radiology, Pathology)
- Prefer to work in larger teams to learn from a greater variety of people and develop in a more sociable environment.

The CAMP structure (see 5.1) is useful to help you think about a wide range of reasons and gives you a natural structure. You can use it as you see fit in relation to your own situation.

You do not have to find one reason in each category; for example, it would be perfectly fine to have two clinical reasons and one management reason; or one clinical reason, one management reason and one personal reason. What matters is that you can present suitable variety in a structured manner.

It is crucial that you remain true to yourself if you want to appear enthusiastic. Not everyone wants to join a specific specialty for academic reasons, so don't force yourself to talk about academic reasons if they do not represent your true motivations. You will only invite further questions which will make you regret having mentioned it in the first place.

Example of an ineffective answer

"I have acquired all the skills to do well in Obstetrics & Gynaecology and I feel that I have a lot to offer the specialty. I also want to train in Obstetrics & Gynaecology because I think it is an interesting and challenging specialty. I like the surgery, I enjoy caring for women and I think that there is no better job than to help a baby enter life."

Why this answer does not work well

This answer is ineffective for several reasons:

- It consists mostly of a list of reasons, with no real attempt to substantiate them. None of the reasons have been developed in any depth. In particular, the use of words such as "interesting" and "challenging" without an explanation of why the specialty is so attractive makes the answer particularly vacuous. Also, what does the candidate mean by "I enjoy caring for women"? What does he/she enjoy about it?

- The candidate does not attempt to link his/her explanations to their experience or personal story. When delivered orally, the answer will sound unenthusiastic and bland. There is a need for more depth, which would in turn translate into a more dynamic answer.

- One of the reasons that the candidate presents is that he/she has the skills for the specialty. The main problem is that we all have skills that would make us suitable for jobs that we don't particularly want to do. Having the skills is therefore not a sign of motivation. These skills may be something worth mentioning in the answer, but only as a conclusion and providing the candidate explains, even if briefly, what these skills are.

On the positive side, there is an attempt to choose a range of reasons which are of a different nature, e.g. a technical reason (liking the surgery), a patient-based reason (enjoying caring for women) and personal satisfaction.

Example of an effective answer

"Obstetrics & Gynaecology is a specialty in which I have developed an interest since my first attachment in Obstetrics at medical school; and which I have learnt to discover and enjoy further during my Foundation Years attachments.

One aspect of the specialty that I have particularly enjoyed is the variety it offers. You can experience extreme joys – for example when helping to deliver babies – but you also have opportunities to help patients through particularly difficult times – for example when dealing with miscarriages or cancers. I personally experienced these highs and lows when I helped an HIV-positive woman safely deliver a healthy baby, whilst the very next day having to console a patient who had just been told that she would need to have an operation that could result in subfertility. I feel very enthusiastic at the prospect of being able to make a difference to women in situations which evoke such extremes of emotions, high or low.

I like the fact that Obstetrics & Gynaecology is a very procedure-based specialty complemented by a challenging medical side. During my attachments, I enjoyed performing examinations and observing procedures such as hysteroscopies, diagnostic laparoscopies and open surgery. I have always thoroughly enjoyed both surgery and medicine, and I feel that a career in Obstetrics & Gynaecology would enable me to develop both interests.

From a personal perspective, I find the holistic approach that Obstetrics & Gynaecology offers very rewarding. Having attended sexual health clinics and women's health clinics both as a medical student and as a junior doctor has really helped

---

me appreciate how much difference we can make in addition to the purely physical needs of the patient. This makes Obstetrics & Gynaecology a well-rounded specialty.

Finally, I feel that the specialty offers a wonderful opportunity to work closely with other members of a team. I have particularly enjoyed the buzz of working on labour wards with midwives and the challenge of ensuring good communication and team working to ensure the safety of our patients, despite the sometimes fast-moving conditions and the possible conflicts that can develop as a result of shared responsibilities."

This answer can be delivered in just over 1½ minutes at normal pace, which should reassure you that a three-point personalised approach works well.

Beware of criticising other specialties

Candidates commonly criticise other training schemes (e.g. explain that they chose medicine because they found surgery too boring or surgery because they found that medicine does not achieve fast results). This would give answers along the lines of: "I feel that surgery can be very samey and that there is no real opportunity for prolonged contact with patients after the follow-up. Medicine, on the other hand, is much more varied and does offer better opportunities for continuity of care."

You can see how inflammatory such an answer could be. And even if the interviewers agree with the candidate, it will no doubt present him/her as someone who is negative. The answer does not sell the candidate's love for medicine in a positive manner. In particular, the lack of examples makes the candidate appear judgemental.

Generally, I would advise against selling your interest for one specialty by putting another one down. You must make sure that you present a positive image. The only exception to this would be if you have changed career path, in which case you could explain your interest in the specialty by comparing it to your previous specialty. If you do this, make sure that you sell the positive points of your previous specialty. When mentioning the negative aspects, present them as something that you did not enjoy rather than generalising with sentences like "Specialty X is not very interesting because ..."

The best format to explain a switch of specialty would be to explain:

- What you enjoyed about your previous
- Why you felt limited within it
- Why this new specialty is the answer to your problems.

Selling your enthusiasm for a Core Training post

Those who are applying to named specialties (e.g. Ophthalmology, Cardiology, O&G, Paediatrics, Anaesthetics, Urology, ENT, etc.) should find it easier to explain their career choice than those applying to Core Training posts. Indeed, those applying to Core Training schemes in medicine, surgery or acute care are not actually applying for a specific specialty and may therefore lack focus in their answer. Specialties within medicine or surgery can be very different from one another and this leads to some candidates sounding vague and seemingly unmotivated.

There are, however, aspects which are common to all or most specialties within medicine, surgery or acute care. Here are a few to get you started:

Medicine
- Excellent problem-solving environment
- Opportunity to deal with psychosocial issues as well as physical
- Good mix of ward and clinic work
- Opportunity to follow up patients with chronic illnesses
- Enjoy contact with patients
- A lot rests on your communication skills
- Enjoy the varied teamwork.

Surgery
- Enjoy manual/technical skills and challenges
- Enjoy the satisfaction of making an immediate difference to patients
- Good mix of acute and chronic patients
- Enjoy the fact that it is very evidence-based and fast moving
- Look forward to research opportunities
- Enjoy working under pressure.

Acute Care
- Enjoy working under pressure
- Enjoy the challenge of dealing with the unexpected
- Strong communication challenge too in terms of reassuring patients and relatives, and managing expectations
- Good teamwork angle, particularly in dealing with other specialists.

You can of course add your own reasons based on your own experience of the field to which you are applying. By following a similar pattern to the answer given earlier, and, more importantly, by using your own experience, you will be able to create a strong answer.

If you already have an idea of the specialty that you want to do once you have completed your Core Training rotation, then I would suggest that you use it in your answer too. However, be careful to only bring it up at the end of the answer (i.e.

your third paragraph). If you go on about one single specialty throughout the whole answer, you will cause three problems:

- The consultants interviewing you will often be from a different specialty and they will be looking for some balance (you wouldn't want to bruise their egos too much...).

- You will give the feeling that you may be bored during the Core Training rotation whenever you are not working in your chosen specialty. This could be problematic if your two-year rotation only contains 4 months in that specialty (if anything).

- By spending the whole answer on one specialty, you may face a secondary question of the type: "What will you do if you don't get into Cardiology in two years' time?"

By spending two paragraphs talking about medicine, surgery or acute care generally and by focusing on your chosen specialty in the final paragraph, you will establish a sensible balance in your answer. This will show that you are motivated for the whole programme but that you also have a clear focus.

Better still, you could identify two specialties which are of a similar nature. For example, Cardiology and Gastroenterology both have a diagnostic and a procedural side. In that way, you do not show too strong a focus on one specialty but you retain your focus in the answer. By mentioning two specialties rather than one, you also present yourself as someone who is open-minded.

So, your third paragraph could be follows:

"Finally, the two specialties that I have particularly enjoyed over the past 3 years have been Cardiology and Gastroenterology because they provide a good mix of pure medicine, including diagnosis and management, and of procedures (for example, pacemaker implantation and endoscopies). Core Medical Training would help me find out more about both specialties so that I can make the right choice."

7.4 Why do you want to train in this region/deanery?

We all know that the real answer to this question is either "Because that's where I live" or "Because that's where there are jobs!" However, the marks for these are likely to be minimal.

What the interviewers are looking for

The marking for this question is fairly consistent across all deaneries. All deaneries will be looking for candidates who are motivated for the training that they offer and will expect you to have developed a good understanding of their training programme (i.e. it is not enough to state geographical reasons for wanting to work or train in a particular region). As well as good reasons, the interviewers will expect good and clear explanations of your motivation. Here is an example of a marking schedule:

0	No clear reason
1	Vague geographical reasons, but no reasons relating to the training programme
2	Limited understanding of the training programme with unclear reasons
3	Reasonable to good understanding of the training programme with clearer reasons
4	Excellent understanding of the training programme. Clear and detailed explanations of the reasons

As you can see, the marking structure leaves some room for subjective judgement but one thing is clear: you should do some homework about the deanery to identify what the training scheme offers; otherwise you will struggle to score more than 2.

For most deaneries, you should be able to score at least 3 by spending a minimum of time reading relevant internet sites or talking to people who are already training there. With a bit more homework and a clear structure, you could easily score the maximum mark. Clearly, this is a question to expect and this simple preparation makes it easy to score well.

What reasons can you mention?

Here again you can use the CAMP structure (see 5.1) to help brainstorm for reasons and structure the answer appropriately.

Clinical reasons (including clinical practice and clinical training)
- The area covers a varied population (e.g. ranging from deprived to affluent populations, multiethnic or otherwise), thus providing a good case mix for training.
- The region covers types of patients that are of particular interest to the specialty applied for (e.g. a primarily elderly population, a strong refugee population, strong diabetes prevalence, etc.).
- The rotation provides training in a mix of different settings (e.g. good exposure to both DGH and tertiary centres, or community settings for some specialties) or, on the contrary, it has more DGH or tertiary exposure (depending on what your future plans are).
- Some of the hospitals are renowned centres for the specialty to which you are applying, thus allowing you better exposure to your future specialty of choice, or special interest that you are interested in developing.
- The deanery provides good support for taking and passing exams, with established structured programmes.
- The deanery encourages and provides support for trainees to pass specialty-specific exams early, which may not be compulsory (a sign that the training programme is attempting to stretch its trainees, which would suit the more ambitious candidates).
- The deanery has achieved high pass rates at Royal College exams, which reflects the quality of support received.

Academic reasons
- The training programme actively encourages an involvement in research.
- You are interested in research and the deanery contains centres which would enable you to further that interest.
- You may already have developed research projects in this region and wish to continue training in the same region to complete or pursue these projects further.
- You have an interest in teaching and will be primarily training in teaching hospitals, thus giving you opportunities to get involved.
- Local medical schools employ teaching methods which match your interest and experience, and with which you will have opportunities to become involved.
- Teaching qualifications are encouraged for those interested.
- The deanery runs good courses for research and teaching.

Management reasons
- The deanery encourages active participation in audit.
- The deanery provides structured management training (e.g. running in-house courses).
- There are opportunities to take on responsibilities (e.g. clinical governance, service development).

Personal reasons
- You have worked/trained in the region before and enjoyed your time there (you should be able to explain what you enjoyed).
- Your wife, husband or partner works in the region.
- Your family, relatives and/or friends are close by, thus providing a good support network.
- You have responsibilities which would warrant working in that region. This could include caring for relatives, social responsibilities, responsibilities with local charities or other associations.
- You enjoy the region.
- You have hobbies or personal interests that would be best maintained in that region.

These are just a few of the reasons that you can discuss and should give you a starting point to think about your own.

One question, which I am often asked, is whether it is acceptable to bring social reasons into the answer. Those who ask are concerned that they may be projecting the wrong image. The answer to this question is that it is acceptable because the right social circumstances are likely to make you a better and more stable trainee. However, you should ensure that social reasons are mentioned at the end of the answer, after you have successfully demonstrated your knowledge of the training programme.

Example of an ineffective answer

"I want to work in the East of England because of the variety of population and the different experiences that I can gain there. It is also close to London where most of my family and friends are based, whilst also providing access to the countryside."

What makes the answer ineffective?

Although the candidate alludes to the variety that the deanery offers, it is not very clear as to what that variety is and why this is relevant to the candidate's training. The answer could be given in just about every deanery in almost every specialty, and it is clear that the candidate has made no effort to research the training scheme that he/she is applying for and to describe why that training scheme is of particular interest. This answer would probably score 1 mark only because it has a strong focus on the geography and personal reasons, but not much else.

Example of an effective answer

"I feel that East of England is an ideal region for Cardiology training, for many reasons.

First of all, it offers a huge variety in terms of settings. There is a good selection of smaller hospitals such as Kings Lynn, Hinchingbrooke and Bury St Edmonds, larger centres such as Addenbrooke's and Norwich, but also specialist tertiary centres such as Papworth. The East of England also covers a vast area, encompassing rural and urban areas from Norwich to Bedford, as well as middle-class and deprived populations. This makes the training scheme very broad-ranging and provides a good opportunity to get involved in all clinical aspects of Cardiology.

I also know from my background reading that many of the hospitals are investing a lot of resources into cardiac services, for example through the creation or increase in capacity of catheter labs in Kings Lynn, Ipswich and Cambridge, some of which will be mobile. This obviously increases opportunities to gain hands-on experience in interventional cardiology (one of my areas of interest) but also demonstrates that the region is forward thinking in its approach, which makes it an exciting environment in which to train.

One of the area's great assets, in my opinion, is also that it contains major teaching hospitals such as Addenbrooke's and Norfolk and Norwich Hospital. The proximity to one of the oldest and one of the newest medical schools provides a unique opportunity for me to become involved in a wide range of teaching activities and to develop new skills, both in traditional teaching methods and in newer ones such as problem-based learning. Working near major centres such as Cambridge and Papworth also makes it an ideal environment to develop research interests.

Finally, so far I have trained mostly in the London area and I am very keen to discover a new environment. The East of England provides a nice semi-rural setting whilst at the same time having the advantage of remaining within easy reach of London, where I have a lot of friends and family.

Overall, I feel that it will provide me with an excellent training in a dynamic environment, both clinically and academically, and will give me many opportunities to develop a strong portfolio which will enable me to give back fully to the specialty once I become a consultant."

This answer can be delivered in approximately 2 minutes. It clearly sets out different reasons in each paragraph, all of which are properly signposted. The candidate has covered several domains including clinical, academic and personal reasons.

The level of detail within each paragraph is just enough to demonstrate that the candidate has seriously considered his reasons and has taken the trouble to do some homework, which is by itself a sign of motivation. More importantly, for each reason, the candidate has demonstrated why it mattered to him. For example, saying that the region was setting up new catheter labs is not interesting by itself until the candidate explains that it will give him an opportunity to gain hands-on experience in interventional cardiology, which is one of his areas of interest. In your answers, make sure that you do not limit yourself to stating a list of reasons; you should explain their relevance to your application.

Finally, the social reasons are highlighted too – though not until the end – to round off the answer and give a more personal dimension.

7.5 Why not train somewhere else?

You may have proudly delivered a good answer to the question "Why do you want to train in this region/deanery?" but there is always someone who will spoil your fun. Whilst question 7.4 was asking you to demonstrate why this region was a good place for you to train, the interviewers now want you to explain why this particular deanery is more attractive than others.

In practice this can be quite tricky to answer because, in many specialties, there isn't much to differentiate one region from the next and the determining factor is often the personal side (i.e. either you have already trained there, you live there, or you have family there). Essentially, there are two possibilities: either you have strong reasons for choosing this region over all others, or they pretty much all look the same to you.

If you have a strong reason

If your reason is making this particular region stand out in relation to the others you should mention it. Reasons that would tie you to a specific region would normally include:

- Having enjoyed training or working there previously
- Having career plans which can only be realised in that area (e.g. in respect of special interests)
- Having academic commitments already started in that region
- Personal responsibilities in the local area (children, other social engagements or responsibilities).

If you do not have a particular reason

If you feel that this particular deanery is only one option amongst several others, you need to take particular care not to come across as disinterested or dismissive. Doctors who work there will want you to show some enthusiasm towards their own deanery and the training that they are delivering. On the other hand, there is no need to pretend that they are a particularly unique deanery if you have no real argument to back that up.

A good way to approach the question in this case is to set out what your criteria for selection are, and to show how the deanery matches. You may also want to reassure them that they are your preferred choice or that you feel they are, overall, stronger than the others, judging for example from the feedback that you have received.

Example of a possible answer

"It is true that there are other regions which look equally interesting; however, ultimately, what I am looking for is a deanery which provides good clinical training in an environment that provides variety and strong support. I also want to train in a deanery that provides good opportunities for research and teaching, and where I will feel comfortable socially.

I think this deanery offers all this and therefore is my preferred choice. In addition, I have talked to colleagues and other people who work here. They are all enjoying their training and the opportunities that they are given to progress so I have absolutely no doubt that I will benefit greatly from training here."

7.6 What is your biggest achievement?

This is a question that gives you the opportunity to impress. The question says "biggest", so stick to one achievement. Mentioning more than one achievement would only dilute the strength of your answer because you would talk superficially about several rather than in-depth about one. You would also be wasting time because the marking scheme will only allow you to score points for one achievement.

This question is not very specific as to what type of achievement the interviewers are looking for. You have a choice between achievements within medicine or outside medicine, academic achievements or non-academic achievements, etc. If you have one particular achievement that you are keen on highlighting, mention that one. If you have several and are unsure as to which they would prefer, then you can ask them what type of achievement they are looking for.

Deriving content for your answer

Use the CAMP structure (see 5.1) to help you derive possible achievements:

Clinical
- Breadth of experience gained
- Progression in training over expectations
- Initiative taken to gain experience in your specialty of choice well beyond basic training requirements
- Prizes or awards at medical school or during your postgraduate training.

Academic
- Substantial involvement in a research project
- Substantial involvement in teaching
- Involvement in the preparation and delivery of an important presentation
- Publication of paper, audit, poster or case report, preferably as 1st author
- Prize for presentation or poster
- Teaching achievements or recognition, e.g. becoming an ALS instructor.

Management
- Substantial involvement in audit or taking charge of an audit which led to important changes in clinical practice
- Successfully managed a rota for a complex team or set-up
- Writing a guideline or protocol.

Personal
- Voluntary work or out-of-programme experience (OOPE)
- Position of responsibility outside of medicine
- Implementing educational website or other key resource
- Having successfully juggled training with difficult personal circumstances
- High achievement in sports, music, arts, etc.

Marking scheme

Marking schemes may vary but they will always centre around the strength of the achievement and the explanation of its significance to you. A typical marking scheme would be as follows:

0	No real achievement
1	Moderate achievement with reasonable explanation of significance
2	High achievement with reasonable explanation of significance or Moderate achievement with clear, detailed explanation of significance
3	Exceptional achievement with reasonable explanation of significance or High achievement with clear, detailed explanation of significance
4	Exceptional achievement with clear, detailed explanation of significance

Nature and strength of the achievement

To produce an effective answer, you must explain clearly not only what the achievement is but also why it is an achievement. This will help the interviewers to mark it as moderate, high or exceptional. The following table is often used by interviewers to determine the level of the achievement:

Exceptional	Less than 10% of your peers would be expected to achieve the same thing or there was a high level of competition.
High	Less than 25% of your peers would be expected to achieve the same thing or there was a reasonable level of competition.
Moderate	Less than 50% of your peers would be expected to achieve the same thing or there was some competition.

You will greatly help the interviewers to mark you well by ensuring that you define how hard you needed to work in order to achieve and/or the level of competition that you faced.

Explanation of the achievement's significance to you

This is an important part of the answer, which is often neglected by candidates. The interviewers will not only want to know that you can achieve, they will also want you to demonstrate that you understand the significance of your achievement and what it says about you.

In your answer, you should therefore highlight why you are particularly proud of your achievement and what can be derived from it. You will also need to make the link back to the post or specialty that you are applying for.

Example 1: Medical school prize

Saying "I got a prize at medical school during my neurology attachment" does not reflect accurately the level of the achievement. The interviewer will not know how hard you needed to work to obtain it or how much competition you faced. Instead you will need to say something along the following lines:

Achievement: "My biggest achievement is a prize that I obtained at medical school for a neurology attachment. I was competing against 30 other students. It involved a written exam and an oral presentation. To achieve the prize I made sure I attended all the teaching sessions and clinics planned, but I also took the initiative to gain further experience by attending extra clinics for neurodegenerative disorders. I also did quite a lot of reading on Alzheimer's and Parkinson's diseases.

Significance: I am particularly proud of the prize because I worked hard to ensure that I was well prepared for the assessment and the reward reflects the interest that I paid to the specialty. In fact one of my reasons for applying to Core Medical Training this year is that I am considering a career either in Neurology or stroke medicine."

This answer is effective because the level of the achievement and effort required are both clearly set out by the candidate. The explanation of the significance is also well developed. The candidate demonstrates why they were proud of the achievement and what it meant to them.

Example 2: Poster presentation

If you consider the answer "During one of my attachments, we had a poster accepted at a regional conference, for which we nearly got a prize", you will see that the impact is minimal. The achievement itself seems exceptional for someone at F2 level; however, the lack of explanation, coupled with the fact that the candidate talks about "we", i.e. the team rather than him/herself, makes it difficult to mark. A better answer would be as follows:

Achievement: "During my F2 attachment in Anaesthetics, I conducted an audit on the availability of difficult airway equipment in obstetrics units, which encompassed results from three major hospitals in the area. The audit highlighted some severe issues, which I summarised in a presentation to my department, following which I was encouraged to write up the audit results as a poster presentation for the <xxx> conference. Not only was my poster accepted for exhibition; it was also selected for an oral presentation, which I gave, and for which I came second overall.

Significance: I am very proud of this achievement for several reasons. Firstly, I played a leading role in the audit and was able to point out some severe failures of the system, which ultimately led to a change in practice and improved patient care. Secondly, being selected for a poster presentation was my first major academic achievement, but being asked to do the presentation really gave me pride in my work. Finally, I was able to put together a good presentation with very little notice, and, although I did not get the first prize, I came close and it really motivated me to get further involved in audits and studies so that I can do even better next time."

This answer works well because we can easily identify the level of involvement and effort made by the candidate. There is sufficient detail without being boring to listen to (for example, the actual results of the audit were missed out deliberately because by themselves they do not form part of the achievement – if the interviewers were interested in the results, they could always ask further questions). The significance of the achievement is also very well laid out, with a good explanation of the motivation gained by the candidate as a result of it.

7.7   What do you like most about this specialty?

The answer to this question can be taken directly from question 7.3 – "Why do you want to train in this specialty?" – as they are effectively the same question. It may be, however, that the interviewers ask you to focus on one specific positive point of the specialty. You can simply pick on one of the points, but this may leave you with a feeling that you are not selling yourself fully. There is a good trick that you can adopt if you want to present several attributes in the same answer without sounding like you are not answering the question properly. Consider this answer:

"There are plenty of aspects that I like about Paediatrics. I enjoy the teamwork element of the specialty, the communication challenge of having to convey similar information at a child and an adult level, as well as the fact that you can deal with a lot of specialties within the course of one day.

However, if I had to isolate one particular aspect of Paediatrics, I would say that, what I enjoy most is that you can really make a strong difference to someone's life and there is nothing that gives me more satisfaction than the smile on a mother's face when she sees that we have made a big difference to her child. It can be very emotional but it is also very rewarding at times. For example, <then talk briefly about a recent situation which illustrates your point>."

If you look closely at the answer, you will see that the candidate has mentioned briefly a few positive features of the specialty, before quickly settling on what he/she regards as the most rewarding. In all fairness, the marking scheme is likely to account only for one positive and therefore, as such, you may not score extra marks for the daring introduction. However, this technique will make your answer much more dynamic. In turn, it will make you sound more enthusiastic and it may well influence the interviewers subconsciously in providing a slightly higher mark. This could be the difference between getting 3 marks for a good answer and 4 marks for an excellent answer.

7.8 What do you like least about this specialty?

The interviewers will be looking for honesty and a realistic insight into the specialty. Here are some examples of points that you can raise:

- Medicine (in general): being given inappropriate referrals. Having to deal with constant demands to discharge patients, sometimes borderline
- Surgery (in general): some aspects of the work may be repetitive
- Paediatrics: it can be emotionally difficult to deal with cases where you know that there is little you can do for a child (and more so for neonates). Dealing with challenging child protection issues
- O&G: dealing with distressing situations such as stillbirths or sexual assaults. Challenging teamwork environment
- Oncology: feeling of powerlessness for some patients. Poor outcomes
- A&E: having to put up with angry or drunk patients or the feeling that sometimes you are dealing with a lot of self-inflicted problems, which deflect attention from other more important matters
- Orthopaedics: some repetitive aspects (e.g. routine hip replacements)
- Respiratory: feeling of fighting a losing battle when dealing with a lot of self-inflicted problems
- Cardiology: dealing with patients with end-stage heart failure for whom treatment options are limited
- Gastroenterology: dealing with patients with more functional/non-organic conditions for which non-invasive investigations are unhelpful and you may have to persuade patients to accept that their symptoms may not be simply cured by a course of tablets or invasive procedure
- Diabetes: can be repetitive unless broken into special interests
- Psychiatry: can sometimes be difficult to retain professional barrier with patient (i.e. not get involved emotionally). For adult psychiatry, feeling that sometimes nothing can be done for a patient any more. Having to deal with stigma attached to psychiatry
- Ophthalmology: repetitive nature of some of the work (e.g. cataracts)
- Radiology: a lot of solo work (e.g. reporting). Having to fight unreasonable requests from other specialists
- Anaesthetics: not in control of the full patient pathway. Many periods of "low demand" where extra vigilance is required
- ENT: dealing with high expectations from patients (e.g. curing snoring).

There are no right or wrong answers. However, in order to optimise the impact of your answer, you will need to consider the following:

- Unless specifically asked, do not mention more than one negative aspect
- You must justify your answer using your experience

- If you can, introduce your answer with one or two quick positive aspects to place the negative into a more neutral context
- Reassure the interviewers that you can deal/cope with this negative and explain how/why.

Example of an effective answer

Positive introduction	"I find it difficult to find something that I don't like in Accident and Emergency because I think that the specialty has a lot to offer both in terms of variety and the personal satisfaction to be able to deal with people at a particularly vulnerable time.
Clear answer	However, there is perhaps one aspect of A&E which I have enjoyed less than others and this is the fact that we sometimes have to deal with patients who have high expectations of a stretched system, even when their injuries are fairly minor and they see that we are busy dealing with real emergencies. Some of our clients don't tend to be very patient and can sometimes become very vocal or abusive.
Illustrative example	For example, a couple of months ago, during my A&E attachment, I dealt with a patient who had a wart on his thumb and should really have gone to his GP. He had become aggressive because he felt he should have been given a higher level of priority. At the time I was able to deal successfully with his behaviour through listening and providing clear explanations for the delays and the prioritisation; but it was frustrating.
Coping with it	I am usually very good at dealing with pressure and I have always been able to handle the more 'hairy' moments appropriately and with good outcomes. One of the reasons I want to do A&E is because I feel that I build a good rapport with people even in challenging circumstances and, in many ways, I am very much looking forward to taking on this challenge."

7.9 What have you done outside of your regular scheduled daily activities that demonstrates your interest in the specialty?

The question is asking for experience that you organised to gain an insight into the specialty. Note that the question precludes you from discussing any activities which formed part of your normal duties. It has to be above your normal duties, i.e. something that you took the initiative to organise or to get involved in.

Finding content for your answer

The list below contains some of the experiences that you can use to sell your interest and commitment:

- Seeking special attachments or "tasters" in the specialty
- Attending relevant teaching sessions (for example, many medics/surgeons attend X-ray meetings; general medics attend oncology MDT meetings; surgeons attend trauma meetings, etc.)
- Undertaking a project in the specialty (e.g. audits, presentations)
- Discussing a possible career in the specialty with a consultant
- Shadowing an SHO/Registrar/ST in your spare time
- Voluntarily sitting in on clinics in that specialty
- Reading up on specialty-related issues (journals, internet sites)
- Attending conferences (specialty associations or other)
- Studying for exams or certificates related to the specialty
- Online CME activities through recognised institutions/websites
- Choosing an elective at medical school which was in that field
- Doing a dissertation for your BSc or otherwise on a related topic.

Think laterally about experience acquired in related specialties

The experience does not have to be in the specialty itself. For example, let's assume that you wanted to apply to Psychiatry. One obvious way to demonstrate your interest in the specialty would be to initiate an audit during a Psychiatry attachment. However, you may also have used your initiative to get involved in Psychiatry-related projects during a General Practice attachment, an Elderly Care attachment, or even an Accident and Emergency attachment.

Similarly, if you are applying for Obstetrics and Gynaecology, you may have volunteered to attend additional theatre sessions during your O&G attachment. You may also have attended specialist clinics in the Genitourinary Medicine department or training sessions with the neonatal team.

Marking schedule

A typical marking schedule would be as follows:

0	No clear evidence
1	Examples are not related to the specialty, or they are but the candidate has not demonstrated the relevance
2	Some evidence provided but it is basic, explanations are relatively vague and relevance to the specialty is not explained
3	One good example provided with relevance to the specialty highlighted, clear explanation of how the candidate developed experience, skills or understanding as a result
4	More than one good example provided, showing relevance to the specialty, clearly explaining how the candidate developed their experience, skills or understanding as a result

From this sample marking schedule, you can clearly see that to maximise your mark you need to provide several relevant examples with full explanation of relevance and personal reflection. Any vagueness in the answer will make you score at most 2 marks, even if you have several items to discuss.

Example of an effective answer (Radiology)

"In addition to my regular discussions with radiologists in the course of all my previous jobs, whether they were in Accident and Emergency, Geriatrics, Cardiology, Intensive Care or Endocrinology, I have also sought many additional opportunities to become involved in radiology audit projects or studies and completed two projects last year under the guidance of a consultant radiologist.
I performed an audit on the complication rate of tunnelled central lines in radiology and did a study that compared ultrasound aided and unaided liver biopsies. Both enabled me to get a good grasp of some of the important issues affecting radiology, particularly on the interventional side.

I have also made every effort to attend courses that would enhance my knowledge. Over the past two years, I have attended four radiology-related courses on topics as diverse as cardiovascular radiological imaging and diagnostic imaging in Emergency Medicine. I am due to attend a further meeting later this year on plain film reporting. Although some of these courses were quite complex, they provided me with a better understanding of some of the issues that I had come across during my A&E and Cardiology posts. They have also shown me the diversity that radiology offers.

Finally I have taken up membership of a number of radiology societies, such as the British Institute of Radiology, the British Society of Skeletal Radiology and the European Congress of Radiology. This gives me access to a range of websites and publications that I consult in my spare time. Like the courses that I attend, it gives me further insight into the specialty. Some of the sites also have online CPD exercises, which I have found useful."

Example of an effective answer (Trauma & Orthopaedics)

"Trauma and Orthopaedics is the surgical specialty that I have most enjoyed over the past few years and, as a result, I have taken the initiative to get involved in many projects in this field.

I have recently taken up a 2-year distance learning MSc with Warwick University, which contains modules such as 'Managing Upper Limb Pain' and 'External Fixators'. I found this course to be an excellent complement to my daily activities as it not only allowed me to continue my training in T&O during other attachments in my rotation, but it also allowed me to consolidate what I learnt on the shop floor.
On top of that, I have made a point of attending several T&O courses. Over the past 3 years, I have attended an average of three courses per year, including the Royal College course on 'Core skills in operative orthopaedics', a course on 'Basic knee arthroscopy' also last year, and the Edinburgh Instructional Trauma Management Course a couple of years ago. These courses have helped me in my daily work and proactively getting involved in Continuing Professional Development will put me in good stead to keep my skills up to date throughout my career.

Finally, I have attended the optional weekly radiology meeting, combined orthopaedics/rheumatology meetings and combined neurosurgical/spinal surgeon meeting. These have been particularly useful in helping me understand the interaction between T&O and other specialties and certainly showed me how much more can be achieved through teamwork, even when there are disagreements."

Example of an effective answer (Genitourinary Medicine)

"During my attachment in respiratory medicine last year, I arranged to sit in on a number of GU and HIV clinics with the local GU consultant. I attended three female GU clinics, two male GU clinics, three HIV clinics and three health advisers' counselling sessions, which gave me an excellent insight into the nature of the clinical problems encountered as well as the intricacies of managing HIV patients. In particular, I gained an appreciation of the ethical issues associated with confidentiality and partner notification.

Last year I did an audit of needle stick injuries amongst hospital staff. Through this audit, I learnt much about risk management and the prescription of post-exposure prophylaxis. It also gave me an opportunity to discover how A&E handles occupational injuries.

Finally, I have attended two conferences, one on Chlamydia and the other on the management of HIV for sex workers, which gave me a good introduction to current issues."

All three examples work well because they contain three key points, which are developed in a personal manner. The candidates stick to the point and avoid waffling. This makes the delivery confident and enables the interviewers to tick the boxes.

7.10 Where do you see yourself in 10 years' time?

This question requires some degree of thought if you don't want to provide an answer of the type "Well, I see myself as a consultant caring for patients", which would be quoting the obvious and would guarantee you a poor mark. Again, you can think along the lines of the CAMP structure (see 5.1) to gather your thoughts and structure your answer:

Clinical

- If you are applying for a Core Training scheme, which specialty would you like to get into? There is no need to focus on one if you can't but try to narrow your preferences a little to your most likely choices. For example, if you are doing CMT, you may not be able to decide which specialty you want to do but you have a preference for those which are partly interventional (e.g. Cardiology, Gastroenterology).
- If you are applying for a specific specialty, are there any particular interests that you want to develop? For example, if you are applying for ST1 Psychiatry, would you be more interested by child and adolescent, adult, learning disabilities, substance misuse subspecialties? If you are applying for Anaesthetics, perhaps you are interested in obstetrics anaesthesia, ITU or pain management.
- You clearly want to be a consultant, but in what type of hospital? Do you want to work in a DGH or a teaching hospital?

Academic

- Are you interested in doing research? If so, why? What makes you say that? Do you already have experience of research? What topics interest you?
- Have you already developed research interests that you are keen to pursue?
- Do you have an interest in teaching that you are keen to develop? What kind of personal development do you envisage undertaking? Do you want to be an ALS instructor? Do you want to get involved at Royal College level? Are there particular areas that you have enjoyed teaching and would like to become further involved in? Do you intend to gain further teaching qualifications (e.g. medical education degree)?

Management

- Do you want to be involved in service development? Perhaps you have had opportunities to get involved in developing guidelines or improving services.
- Are you interested in managing and supervising others, for example by becoming an educational supervisor?
- Are you interested in developing training programmes?
- Do you have an interest in some aspects of governance in which you would like to become involved (e.g. patient information, risk management).

- In 10 years' time you won't have had a chance to become clinical director, but you could look slightly further and determine whether you are keen to develop management responsibilities further down the line.

Personal
- Which type of region do you see yourself working in?
- What type of team do you see yourself being part of?
- Responsibilities outside work (charity, voluntary work).
- Hobbies.

Example of an effective answer (for ST1 surgery)

"Ten years time is a long way away but, certainly, by that time I will have completed my training and become a consultant. So far, I have particularly enjoyed working in DGHs because you are often dealing with a high turnover of patients and deal with a wide spectrum of problems and this is therefore the setting in which I see myself working in the long term. Clinically, I will have the opportunity through my core surgical training to determine which specialty I enjoy most; however, so far, the two specialties that I have been very keen on are urology and GI surgery. Both have a strong laparoscopic side which I enjoy and both also have the strong research element that I am looking for in my career.

Over the past couple of years, I have really enjoyed participating in teaching programmes, whether by giving lectures to medical students, running revision workshops for finals or even simply mentoring juniors and students on the job. This is certainly an avenue that I am keen to develop and to achieve this I am keen to attend a number of teaching courses and perhaps also do a medical education degree. I know that these degrees can be quite onerous time-wise and therefore I think it would be a good idea if I started doing it earlier in my career rather than when I get too close to my CCT date to give it the time it deserves. From a more personal perspective, I am involved outside of work in voluntary work, teaching disadvantaged children at a local school and raising funds for a charity which sends medical equipment to African countries and I would hope that I get sufficient time to continue my involvement either with these institutions or others of a similar nature."

This answer works well because:
- It goes beyond the obvious and demonstrates that the candidate has put some thought into his career and motivation.
- It has three points clearly signposted and expanded upon.
- It covers a range of activities (clinical, teaching, voluntary work).

Note also the nice touch brought into the answer by the recognition that doing a medical education degree is hard work (in fact many people give up before they complete them). It is this type of sentence which clearly demonstrates that the candidate has done his homework.

7.11 What skills do you need to improve?

It would be easy to provide an answer such as "I feel that my training has been excellent so far and therefore there is nothing that I need to improve." However, this would score low because, in actual fact, the question aims to determine whether you have any insight into your own skills and attributes, and whether you are proactive in seeking ways to improve. Importantly, the question does not refer to new skills that you want to gain in future, but to existing skills that you need to improve. The distinction is important if you want to avoid going off topic.

Brainstorming for ideas

To think about different topics that you could raise, use the CAMP structure (see 5.1):

Clinical
- Are there procedures that you need to perfect?
- Did you miss out on opportunities to develop exposure to some conditions or procedures either because you were busy building other parts of your CV or because the hospitals in which you rotated did not have a sufficient number of patients on whom you could train?
- Are there areas of clinical practice that could be consolidated or improved by going to formal courses or attending special clinics?

Academic
- Have you been involved in research and struggled with some aspects of it? Perhaps you have not done any research yet, have gained research-related skills on an ad hoc basis, and want to formalise your learning?
- Have you got any teaching experience and want to develop certain aspects of it? Are there aspects of teaching or presentation skills that you need to improve (e.g. speaking to large audiences, or learning to make your teaching sessions more interactive)?

Management
- Did you wish you had done more audits?
- Did you miss out on management opportunities such as organising rotas?
- Have you found it hard sometimes to deal with the complexity of project management?
- Have you found it difficult to negotiate your way out of difficult situations and need to develop more confidence (e.g. getting people to radiology or ITU)?
- Have you found it difficult to find your place in MDT meetings and you need to gain more confidence and assertiveness?

Personal

- Are there interpersonal skills you wish you could have had more formal training in?

Answering the question

There is therefore no need to be too negative about your training. You must be proud of whatever you have done so far and be honest about your areas of weakness. Overall you want to convey that everything went well, but that there are some minor areas which you could have handled differently. The answer could be structured as follows:

- Explain that you really enjoyed your training and why
- State clearly the area that you feel could have been handled differently
- Explain how you feel you should have handled it
- Explain how you plan to correct this in the forthcoming years.

Example of an effective answer

"I feel that my training to date has been extremely good. As well as developing good clinical practice and judgement, I have also built a good portfolio of audits, teaching experience and research exposure, including one publication. The one area which I feel I have not had much opportunity to develop is my management skills. Although I have been involved in a number of projects such as <x, y and z>, where I was able to demonstrate good leadership, I feel that the lack of formal management training and the fact that we constantly rotate between jobs makes it difficult to consolidate all the skills learnt on the job.

I have tried to counter this by having discussions and informal training with my educational supervisor, but I would benefit more by being involved in more long-term projects and attending formal training. As soon as I start my ST3 training, I plan to raise the issue with my consultants so that I can plan my career well ahead in that respect. I would hope to improve this by continuing my interest at work and by attending an appropriate management course."

Another example of an effective answer

"During the course of my training so far I have been heavily developing my audit and teaching portfolio, which has enabled me to learn an awful lot about service improvement, training and communication skills. However, as a result, I have not had much time to undertake research work. I know that as a trainee it is important to develop research skills in order to understand the evidence that we base our practice on. As such, I am keen to develop my understanding of research further. I plan to achieve this by attending and organising journal clubs but also by enrolling myself on courses on topics such as research methodologies. I am also keen to write and publish a paper in my next job."

8 Skills-based questions

Skills-based questions form a substantial part of the bank of those asked at interviews. They can take the form of asking about generic personal attributes such as communication, leadership skills, and team playing. They often also require you to provide specific examples where you demonstrated these skills.

Most candidates tend to neglect these questions during their preparation for interviews, either because they feel they can "wing it" or because they are unsure as to how the questions should be approached, preferring instead to bury their head in the sand, hoping that some of the awkward questions such as "What is your main weakness?" won't come up. The scores on these questions more commonly reflect this lack of preparation – therefore this represents a real opportunity for you to gain points that will separate you from the crowd.

In truth, generic questions can be very difficult to handle at an interview if you have not thought your answers through prior to the big day. I would, therefore, encourage you to spend some time organising your thoughts on the matters raised in this chapter.

8.1 | How would you describe your communication skills?

What is communication and what are they looking for?

The interviewers will be looking for an answer which is mature, relevant to the specialty that you are applying for and backed up with personal examples. To score highly, you must present different facets of your communication skills, demonstrate their relevance to the specialty and provide suitable examples.

Communication is an integral part of your daily working life and is the cement that ensures that you maintain good relationships and that you are effective in your work. In the course of your work, you generally demonstrate the following communication skills:

Active listening and empathy

Active listening and empathy are ways of letting the other person know that you understand their feelings, that you care about what they are saying and that you are non-judgemental.

In your dealings with others, this will translate into the following behaviours:
- Knowing when to keep silent and let the other person speak
- Not interrupting
- Being attentive to what the other person is saying and showing it (open posture, appropriate nodding and good eye contact)
- Probing in a supportive manner and using open questions
- Showing support, warmth, care and attention
- Being sensitive to the emotions of others.

You can demonstrate such behaviours in the following situations:
- Breaking bad news
- Talking to an upset patient, relative or colleague
- Dealing with an angry person (patient or colleague)
- Handling complaints
- Dealing with a conflict
- Discussing problems with colleagues (work-related or personal).

As a result, you will achieve the following:
- Gain cooperation from the other person
- Build trust and develop a rapport
- Make people feel more confident
- Encourage discussion and greater openness.

Conveying information in a clear and structured manner

As a doctor, you need to convey your message in a manner that suits your audience. In practice, this will include the following behaviours:
- Anticipating the needs of your audience
- Using clear and unambiguous language, with appropriate jargon
- Choosing the most appropriate communication method, e.g. written, face-to-face, telephone, email, models, diagrams, leaflets
- Adapting your communication to the understanding of your audience.

You can demonstrate such behaviours in the following situations:
- Explaining procedures or management plans to patients
- Seeking consent
- Writing discharge summaries, reports or notes
- Presenting a patient to a senior colleague with a view to gaining advice
- Teaching colleagues
- Presenting at a meeting
- Educating a patient about a chronic condition, or writing leaflets.

As a result, you will achieve the following:
- Better cooperation and appropriate response from the other person
- Time efficiency
- Fewer mistakes/errors.

Influencing and negotiating skills

During the course of your daily work, you will be confronted by difficult situations, disagreements, or even conflicts. To resolve them, you will need to influence other people (i.e. make sure that they do what you want them to do without coercing them or manipulating them, which could aggravate the situation and build resentment).

You will also need to negotiate. In your dealings with others, this will translate into the following behaviours:
- Understanding the impact of your communication on others and adapting your approach accordingly
- Confidently but non-aggressively setting out and defending your point of view
- Being tactful and diplomatic
- Being encouraging and constructive when talking to others.

You can demonstrate such behaviours in the following situations:
- Dealing with a difficult colleague (e.g. not pulling his/her weight)
- Dealing with difficult patients or complaints
- Conflicts with nurses/midwives or any other colleague
- Conflict within an MDT environment due to different personal agendas

- Negotiating the admission of a patient onto a different ward (e.g. if doing general on-calls) or into ITU
- Designing rotas
- Negotiating study or annual leave.

As a result, you will achieve:
- Outcomes that match your expectations
- Better working relationships and understanding of your colleagues.

Answering the question

To produce an effective answer, you need to reflect on your day-to-day experiences and determine in which context you have used the above skills. You only need to discuss a small number of points but it is important that these points are backed up by your personal experience. The answer must be *your* answer and not some standard explanation of what constitutes communication skills.

Blow your own trumpet. At an interview, you must sell yourself positively; it would make no sense to play down your communication skills. Even if you think that you are not that good, you need to find the courage to state that you are; if you don't sell yourself, the interviewers won't be doing it for you!

Phrases to avoid:
- "My communication skills are above average" (not very positive)
- "My communication skills are okay" (meaningless and uninspiring)
- "My communication skills could be improved" (are they bad?)
- "I would give myself 8 out of 10 (meaningless; why not 9 or 10?)
- "I think that I have good communication skills", if delivered in a sceptical voice (if delivered confidently, it could be okay)
- "My communication skills are excellent" (don't overdo it!)
- "My English could be improved" (They will be testing your English at the interview. No need to shoot yourself in the foot by reminding them of a potential weakness)
- "I am a good communicator because I can speak 5 languages" (the fact that you can speak several languages doesn't mean that you can communicate; there are plenty of people who speak English perfectly and are not good communicators. Of more relevance will be your ability to relate to people at different levels, including those from other cultures or ethnic backgrounds. Languages are only tools that help you achieve this).

Good phrases to use:
- "I have good communication skills"
- "My communication skills are very good"
- "I have developed good communication skills" (this recognises that communication is an evolving skill)

- "I have effective communication skills" (meaning that they are achieving results – it saves you having to say that you are good)
- "I have received very positive feedback on my communication skills, not only from nurses and other colleagues, but also from patients" (Remember: feedback is a good way to introduce objectivity in your answers).

Many candidates feel uneasy saying that they are good. This unease comes from the tendency to limit their answer to a single statement of the type "I feel that I have good communication skills" which, if not backed up by concrete examples, will sound very boastful and arrogant. Your answers can sound genuine only if you mention practical examples; by being down to earth and practical, you will reach your comfort zone, which in turn will make you feel more confident in your delivery. Mentioning feedback received will also help make your answers more realistic and will make you sound and feel more confident.

Example of an ineffective answer (commonly given)

"I think that my communications skills are okay but obviously can be improved. Communication is particularly important in my specialty because we have to discuss complex issues with patients and be able to talk to them in a way they understand. We also have to break bad news and deal with difficult patients. I can speak several languages including English, Hindu and Tamil, which can be extremely useful in the region where I work, and I have also done a lot of teaching, which is also important in the specialty."

On the positive side, the candidate has attempted to discuss a variety of communication issues. However, this answer is ineffective because:

- The candidate focuses on tasks (breaking bad news, teaching) and not on skills so much: the skills which enable him/her to carry out these tasks effectively (e.g. empathy, listening, etc.).
- The answer discusses the importance of communication more than the candidate's abilities to communicate.
- The candidate does not sell him/herself (e.g. "okay").
- The candidate uses words which are detached (e.g. "in my specialty"). If you are applying to a given specialty, then why not mention its name? Stating "Communication is particularly important in Ophthalmology" (say) would be more effective. Similarly, if you come from abroad, do not say "In my country", but "In India", or "In Poland, where I first trained". It makes the answer more personal and more direct.
- Listing English as a language is not relevant. As for the other languages, they do not indicate that the candidate can communicate; merely that he has tools to perhaps relate to patients from certain ethnicities. The link between the languages and how they demonstrate a good ability to communicate should be made more explicit.

- Stating that the skills "obviously can be improved" is a reasonable statement to make; however, mentioned in this manner, it suggests that the candidate is not very good at communication. Instead, the candidate should convey a more positive message by mentioning that he/she is constantly finding opportunities to develop his/her communication skills further (for example, by attending courses such as a recent teaching course). This would create a more positive feeling.

Example of an effective answer

"Throughout my training I have developed effective communication skills across a wide range of areas. One of my main strengths is my ability to relate to others and empathise with them. During my diabetes attachment, I often dealt with patients who felt very apprehensive and at times overwhelmed by their diagnosis, its potential complications and implications. I found I could easily engage with them at a level where they felt comfortable expressing their thoughts and feelings. I can remember a couple of patients who had been particularly affected because of the impact of diabetes on their lifestyle, and who commented later that they felt I had given them the time they needed to deal with the issues that mattered to them. They felt that my communication approach helped them to open up.

As well as this, I feel comfortable expressing my opinions clearly in the different areas of work. I take great care to prepare well to ensure that I don't miss any important points and I take account of what other people want to know and of what they will be doing with the information. For instance, on a ward round, I ensure that I focus on the salient points and leave aside the unimportant details. When discussing a diagnosis or treatment plan with a patient, I ensure that I take account of their prior knowledge. I can then convey information that I feel will matter to them.

Over the course of my training so far, I have developed good negotiation and influencing skills. Experience has taught me how everyone in a working system has their own priorities, pressures and even agendas. I feel that, as I have developed an increased clinical understanding, I have improved my ability to prioritise my patients' needs against those of colleagues. This means that I am better able to judge whether to push for something in the interest of my patient or, perhaps, having listened to my colleague, allow them to take priority - for example, when ITU are reluctant to admit a patient or when a radiologist is refusing to perform a scan. I have also learnt to appreciate that not all colleagues respond in the same way even if I try to maintain the same approach, tone and language when dealing with them. One of the lessons that I have learnt as a junior doctor is the importance of remaining calm when dealing with someone who disagrees with you and to try to see things from their point of view. By telling myself that their refusal is nothing personal and by trying to understand their agenda, I have found that I could have very constructive discussions which often led to positive outcomes. In my training in respiratory medicine, this will come in particularly handy."

8.2	**Give an example of a situation where you showed empathy towards a patient**

What situations can you describe?

A good example would be a situation where a patient wanted to take a course of action which you felt was obviously against their best interests. This could include:

- A patient who wanted to self-discharge against medical advice
- A patient who was scared of surgery or a procedure
- A patient who refused to comply with their treatment, condemning themselves to a poor outcome
- A patient who refused to involve relatives but who required strong social and moral support.

Whatever example you choose to describe, you must ensure that it is *your* communication skills that made a difference. You must also ensure that you are not seen to coerce the patient into making a decision.

Answering the question

Since this is a question asking for a specific example, you should use the STAR technique (see 5.2).

Example of an effective answer	
Situation/Task	"Whilst working in Accident and Emergency I saw a young Asian woman who was 6 months pregnant. She was very timid but also appeared to be quite distressed and I felt that she would need some support
Action	To ensure that she had some privacy and felt more at ease, I took her to a cubicle where we could talk more easily. I took my time, made sure that I did not rush her and started to take a history. I could see that she was becoming a little tearful and so used a softer tone of voice. I could see from her composure and her body language that she wanted to tell me more but was somehow reluctant to do so. I felt it was important to let her talk to me in her own time and I gently asked about why she was so upset, reassuring her that it was okay to discuss her feelings. This prompted a sudden release of her emotions, and she started to cry. I gave her some more time to compose herself, making sure that I remained silent in order not to overburden her with words. After a few minutes of silence, she explained that she had miscarried twice before and that her husband and his

	family thought she was an unfit wife. I felt that she was relieved to confide in someone.
Result /Reflect	Once she had opened up we spent some time discussing how she was handling the bottling up of her emotions and I offered her the possibility to see a counsellor if she felt she needed one. Her medical complaint turned out to be minor and with the good rapport we had built she trusted the diagnosis. Overall I found that by listening actively, preparing the scene and mirroring her pace I was able to engage with the patient quickly. Using words that were non-threatening and from her own vocabulary also helped greatly."

This story describes in some detail how the doctor approached the patient and how he made a difference. In this example there are further opportunities to demonstrate empathy by discussing how the doctor then handled the patient once she had admitted what the problem was, but this would make the answer far too long and it may be best to wait to be prompted for more information. Note the reflective paragraph at the end where the candidate states what he/she did well.

8.3 Describe a time when you had to defend your own beliefs regarding the treatment of a patient

What the question is testing and what the interviewers are looking for

The interviewers will be looking for a range of skills including:

- Your ability to listen and take on board criticism without losing your cool
- Your ability to set out your opinions in a constructive manner
- Your ability to influence others in a non-threatening manner.

Scenarios you can discuss

Hopefully this is not a situation that recurs much in your daily working life, so any situation where this has occurred should stand out in your mind. This could be for example:

- A situation where you made a decision that was queried by one of your peers, or seniors or a nurse, and where you had to defend your views
- A situation where your decision or belief with regard to treatment was queried either by the patient or one of his/her relatives
- A case review meeting where you were asked to justify your actions.

How would you normally seek to convince someone that you are right?

- Firstly, you would ensure that you have all the information to hand to be able to present a sensible case.

- Secondly, you would present logical arguments to the other person and would wait for their reaction. You would then pay attention to what they have to say, giving them the opportunity to express their opinion freely without interruption. It will make them feel valued and, you never know, they may have a valid point.

- Thirdly, if your first approach did not work, you may want to try a different approach. In some cases, the alternative approach may be to involve a senior colleague in the debate to give more authority to your argument.

- If none of this works then there may not be an easy conclusion to the problem. If patients are involved, the complaint procedure may need to be invoked or even court action, etc. For the purpose of answering this question you should ensure that you choose an example where you were successful at defending your beliefs otherwise you will run into trouble, however justified your actions were.

Example of an effective answer

Situation/Task   "I had admitted a patient for diabetic ketoacidosis who, I felt, required a high dose of insulin. I asked a staff nurse to administer the treatment, which she refused to do since this was a high dose, beyond that normally given, and she would only give a lower dose.

Action   I spent a couple of minutes explaining patiently and in a normal tone of voice to the nurse, that as well as the patient's blood sugar we needed to deal with the metabolic acidosis, which requires a higher dose of insulin. As she refused to go ahead and, in view of the urgency of the situation, I administered the treatment myself in order to ensure the patient was safe at all times.

Once the patient was stabilised, I asked the nurse if she wanted to discuss the matter in a more relaxed setting. We went to the mess and I asked her to tell me how she saw the situation. She explained that she had never come across a situation like this in her experience and did not feel comfortable giving a potentially dangerous treatment without understanding why.

With her agreement I spent some time explaining the pathophysiology of diabetic ketoacidosis and why a high dose was necessary. I made sure that I kept to terms that she was happy with and throughout our conversation asked her questions to check that I was communicating clearly. I also explained to her in a non-judgemental manner how her actions may have endangered the patient, emphasising that this should in no way stop her from raising her concerns if she felt she needed to in future. Although her behaviour had potentially threatened a patient's health, I wanted to make sure that she used this mistake as a learning point and that we continued to have a good working relationship. To that end, whilst suitably conveying my concerns to her, I made sure that I did not give her a guilt trip.

Result/Reflect   The nurse felt that she understood the situation better and apologised for her action. This incident enabled us to have a closer relationship and, as a result, enhanced the standard of care that we were able to provide to all future patients."

Note the emphasis on the communication aspect of the scenario about listening, being non-judgemental but also assertive. Also note that there is some clinical content; however, it has been reduced to what is strictly necessary to understand the context and the actions of the individuals involved.

Don't be afraid to go into some detail. Detail and facts will help build up your credibility and will make the example look real. But always make sure that those details are relevant to the question being asked.

You can use the "Result/Reflect" section to explain a little bit more than what happened at the end of the story, by adding a sentence about how it helped you become a better doctor. In this example, it is about building bridges with the nurse and enhancing the working relationship. It helps add depth to the answer.

Other questions looking for similar types of answers include: "Give an example of a situation at work where a patient has not agreed with your diagnosis or management."

| 8.4 | **Describe a time when your communication skills made a difference to the outcome of patient care** |

What examples can you use?

The question focuses not just on your communication skills, but on a situation where they actually made a difference to the care of a patient. There are a number of areas that you can explore:

- Situations where the patient was reluctant to agree to a procedure because, perhaps, they were scared (maybe due to a previous bad experience) or had trouble understanding what it involved
- Situations where the patient had needs which they had not clearly expressed and which you managed to identify through good communication
- Situations where you communicated well with a range of members of your team, which then led to efficient action towards the care of a patient.

Although the question does not specify whether the communication skills should be directed towards the patient or towards the team, I would recommend that you play safe by addressing communication with the patient (i.e. the first two points) rather than with the team as this is likely to have a greater impact.

Example of an effective answer

Situation/Task | "Whilst working in Accident and Emergency, an elderly lady presented with left ventricular failure. On being told that she would require admission she became very unhappy and refused to be admitted. After her initial emergency care, I spent some time with her in order to ascertain why she was so reluctant to come in and it transpired that her husband, who was disabled as a result of stroke and dementia, was on his own at home and that she did not want to leave him by himself.

Action | I spent some time listening to the patient and trying to show as much empathy as possible so that I could gain her trust. My main aim at that stage was to let her talk so that I could identify how we could compromise with her.

I explained to her that we would do our utmost to take care of her husband as well as her, and that one solution would be to involve social services so that her husband would be looked after whilst she was recovering. At first she was reluctant to involve social services because she felt that her husband may be taken away from her. I was able to reassure her that this

	would not be the case and that her husband would be well looked after.
Result:	The patient was happy with this solution and subsequently accepted to be admitted.
Reflect:	I felt that I was able to make a real difference by showing real empathy towards the patient at a difficult time for her, and by looking at the situation as a whole rather than concentrating solely on her physical needs."

This example is effective because the story is easy to follow. The context is set out clearly, as is the action that the candidate took. Note the small amount of clinical information, which is just enough to aid the comprehension of the scenario without overwhelming the interviewer with unnecessary detail that would distract from the candidate's communication skills.

The final paragraph summarises the main points that the candidate wishes the interviewers to take on board, effectively highlighting how the example given actually answers the question.

8.5 Give an example of a situation where you failed to communicate appropriately

What the interviewers are looking for

This is a question about learning from a communication mistake. The interviewers will be looking for:

- Honesty in acknowledging your mistake (i.e. professionalism and integrity)
- Sensitive and constructive resolution of the problem at the time
- Ability to reflect, learn from your mistake and change your behaviour

When you are asked to incriminate yourself by describing a situation where you failed to act properly, you should avoid fobbing the panel off with comments such as "I can't remember a situation where I did not communicate well because I always do my best to ensure that I provide the best possible care to my patients". This would actually be missing the point of the question.

What examples can you describe?

You can use examples that relate to patients and relatives as well as other team members. This may include:

- Using unnecessary jargon with a patient
- Being too concise in giving instructions to a junior or to a nurse, not appreciating they may not understand you fully
- Assuming a patient is okay with a particular issue and adopting a normal communication approach, when in fact the patient is actually worried and anxious
- Forgetting to give important information to a colleague, which results in a delay in patient care or discharge
- Complaining to a colleague about their behaviour in an abrupt manner, leading to a conflict
- Being insensitive to someone else's point of view in a meeting, leading to a confrontation
- Dealing with a problem via email or a third party when you would have been better off talking to the person face to face or at least on the phone.

The most powerful answers are those based on real and complex problems. If you choose to talk about an insignificant problem, you will not have much to learn from the scenario and will end up with a weak answer. So, be prepared to take risks if you want to score highly.

How do you deal with the problem?

The way in which you would handle the matter would obviously depend on the nature of the problem. For example:

- If your mistake resulted in a patient not adhering to treatment or a colleague doing the wrong thing because they misunderstood you, then you will need to make sure that you apologise to the patient or colleague and then explain things again in a better manner.
- If your mistake resulted in a confrontation, then you will need to explain how you recognised from their response that you had mishandled the situation, that you apologised and then you corrected the problem by explaining things differently.
- If you were insensitive to someone's point of view at a meeting, you ought to go and see them face to face after the event to apologise and build bridges.

Whatever you did, make sure that you go into enough detail to enable the interviewers to understand that you took the problem seriously and were proactive in resolving the issue.

If the communication problem interfered at any time with patient safety (for example, by delaying treatment because you gave ambiguous instructions), then you must also explain that you took immediate steps to ensure that the patient did not suffer.

Reflect and learn

Once you have described your mistake and how you remedied the situation, reflect on the issues it raises by explaining what you learnt and how you changed your practice thereafter. For example:

"This scenario showed me how important it is to take the time to check the patient's understanding, even if they seem to have understood, as in this case I would have identified straight away that the patient had not fully grasped the impact of the treatment on their lifestyle. The patient was never at risk but getting the communication right would have avoided having to call the patient back for further explanation. I now ensure that I systematically check their understanding throughout the consultation."

8.6	Tell us about a situation where you had to obtain informed consent from a patient who was in a vulnerable situation

This looks like a question on how to seek consent so most candidates would rush into describing how they can seek consent (explain advantages and risks, check the person's understanding, etc.). However, the question is about much more than that. It specifically relates to a vulnerable patient and therefore will be testing the sensitivity of your approach and your ability to recognise and adapt to the patient's specific needs.

Identify vulnerable patients you have encountered

This could include:
- Patients who are elderly, of sound mind but easily influenced
- Patients who may be making decisions against their own best interest because of other factors (e.g. fear of becoming a burden on relatives)
- Patients who have just had bad news broken to them
- Patients who have psychiatric problems.

Answering the question

Here again, the STAR system (see 5.2) will help you.

- Start by explaining the context. Who was the patient (ensuring you give enough detail to show how/why they were vulnerable) and what did you need to seek their consent for?

- Detail how you sought consent (explaining things slowly, checking their understanding, drawing diagrams if needed, etc.) but throughout your answer explain how their vulnerability impacted on your actions and how you resolved each problem that this presented you with. For example, simply saying "I explained the procedure in simple terms" is too weak because this could apply to anyone, not just a vulnerable patient. Instead you could say something along the lines of "I explained the procedure in simple terms, using a diagram to illustrate my words, but the patient seemed a bit confused about some of the detail and was taking a long time to understand some of the basic information. I therefore asked the nurse and also one of the relatives to explain in their own words what I had described, which helped the patient along. Following our explanation I asked the patient to tell me in their own words what they thought was going to happen to them. I also made sure that they had an opportunity to ask questions."

- As another example, instead of saying "the patient was crying so I gave her some leaflets and asked her to come back later", which sounds harsh, you need to explain why you acted in that way and show that you used a sensitive approach that matched the distress of the patient. This could give an answer like "As the patient was crying uncontrollably, I spent some time gently reassuring her that we would do our best for her and asked her if she was okay to continue or wanted to go home. I offered her the opportunity to study some leaflets and come back at a later stage, which she gratefully accepted. She returned three days later, etc."

- Try not to be too technical when explaining how you are seeking consent from the patient as it is not really the aim of the question (which is how you deal with a vulnerable patient). The only really important consent-seeking aspects for this question are:

    - Explaining the procedure in detail in a clear manner, including pros, cons, alternatives, risks (no need to go into detail in these questions)
    - Checking the understanding of the patient and answering their questions
    - Reassuring the patient they can change their mind and can take the time to think about their decision.

In your example, if you have any doubt about the patient's competence then make sure that you explain how you sought to check whether they were competent or not (e.g. by calling for help from a consultant or a psychiatrist). For comprehensive information on patient competence, see Chapter 11.

8.7 | What makes you a good team player?

Before you can answer this question, you must understand what being a team player means. Most candidates are able to quote a few of the attributes of a good team player (the most popular one being that a team player understands his role in the team) but they are unable to explain what they mean in practice. This then makes it difficult to provide meaningful examples.

The following table sets out and develops the key attributes of a good team player. It will help you crystallise your thoughts and come up with your own ideas and examples:

Qualities of a good team player

Understands their role in the team and how it fits within the whole picture
A good team player understands what is expected of him/her and is able to anticipate and address the needs of other members of the team. He/she must also understand what is expected of others so he/she can work with them effectively. In practice, he/she:

- Is reliable, i.e. delivers quality results in a timely manner and follows through on his assignments
- Is consistent, i.e. delivers good quality of work all the time and not just when someone is watching him/her.
- Works hard and does his/her fair share of the work. Takes responsibility to prioritise and organise his/her work appropriately to deliver results
- Involves others appropriately, e.g. asking for advice or help, referring specific issues to others who have greater knowledge of the problem
- Takes the initiative and works as a problem solver, i.e. does not simply do what they are told, does not blame others, does not avoid getting involved and does not let others deal with problems alone.
- Shows commitment to the team. Puts the team's success before his/her own pride/success (e.g. if invited to do a non-glamorous task).

Treats others with respect and is supportive and willing to help
A good team player is considerate and courteous towards their colleagues. He/she demonstrates understanding and shows appropriate support towards others to help get the job done. An effective team player deals with other people in a professional manner.

In practice, he/she:
- Is consistently approachable (i.e. not just when it suits them)
- Responds to others' requests for help, even if it can be inconvenient
- Takes the initiative to offer help when he/she feels someone needs it

- Allows others to express their opinions and respects them
- Takes into account other people's agendas and feelings
- Goes beyond their differences with others and finds ways to work together to get the job done
- Shows diplomacy and tact
- Does not gossip maliciously or attempt to undermine others
- Demonstrates a good sense of humour and knows how to interact with others in a more social context.

Is flexible and adaptable and can compromise
A good team player adapts to ever-changing situations without complaining or resisting. In practice, he/she:

- Can consider different points of view and compromise when needed
- Does not hold rigidly to a point of view especially when the team needs to move forward to make a decision or get on with things
- Is able to strike a compromise between holding on to his/her own beliefs and convictions whilst respecting and taking on board others' opinions
- Shows willingness to change working methods to adapt to new circumstances, without complaining, getting stressed or resisting change.

Communicates constructively and listens actively
Communication is the lynchpin of any good team and a good team player encourages and contributes to good communication. In practice, he/she:

- Speaks up and expresses his/her thoughts and ideas clearly, directly, honestly, and with respect for others and for the work of the team
- Proposes ideas that help resolve problems rather than create them
- Absorbs, understands, and considers ideas and points of view from other people without debating and arguing every point
- Avoids interrupting others to force their point through
- Is willing to accept and listen to comments or criticisms from others without reacting defensively, even if they come from more junior colleagues
- Shares appropriate information with colleagues and keeps them up to date about progress on his/her assignments.

Answering the question

It would be tempting to list all the above qualities in one answer. However, it would sound corny. To answer the question effectively, you must pick three or four of the above skills, which you feel characterise you best, and expand on each using your past experiences. Spreading three points over 2 minutes makes it 40 seconds per point, which gives plenty of time for a couple of brief examples.

Example of an effective answer

"One of my key strengths as a team player is definitely my ability to motivate other people when things are not going well and to support them through hard work and by making myself available to help when required. Over the past 4 months, during my attachment in Oncology, I worked with a couple of other junior doctors. One of them was finding it difficult to come to terms with the terminal aspect of some cancers and I tried to spend some time with her to help her see the positive aspects of our job. I also tried to encourage her to seek some advice from senior colleagues and occupational health, which she did.

As a member of the team I work very hard to ensure that I do all my jobs on time and with the quality that my colleagues expect of me. For example, I work hard to ensure that everything is organised and ready for the morning ward round and that all test results are ready to be presented to the Registrar or consultant. Once the ward round is finished I organise the jobs on a spreadsheet and ensure that I order the appropriate investigations early so that the results are back in time to be checked and acted upon within the working day. In some cases, this involves negotiating with the lab or other colleagues for some urgent review and, when that happens, I ensure that they understand I am trying to get things done with good reason and not simply to impose on their service. I have found that, by remaining calm and polite, I am able to get the majority of tasks done. I have learnt the importance of presenting a good clinical case and not simply arguing when someone shows scepticism.

Finally, I have always been very proactive in discussing problems with colleagues so that we can all improve and the team can provide a better service. As an example, recently I felt that the team had started to become a little inefficient and that the standard of note keeping had gone down. This meant that some investigations were either overlooked or patients were seen twice for no reason. I addressed the issue at a team meeting and offered to do an audit, which has now led to a tightening up of our procedures. By presenting the problem as something that concerned us all rather than by placing the blame on some individuals, I managed to engage the team in resolving the issue."

This answer is effective because it focuses on a handful of key points (i.e. it does not simply list 20 attributes of a good team player); each point is clearly backed up with personal experience and presents the candidate as someone who is clearly playing an active role in the team rather than waiting for others to tell him what to do, when to do it and how to do it.

Warning on mentioning leadership in a "team player" answer

A large proportion of candidates rush to mention that they are good team players because they can both work in a team and be a leader. Leadership is a totally different skill to team playing and you should really avoid mentioning it in an answer to a question that relates to team playing only. In fact, there have been interviews where candidates were told to differentiate between the two (the question was "What makes you a good team player (not a team leader)?"

If you intend to mention leadership (i.e. you don't feel that your answer will be any good without it) then you can do so but you must ensure that it does not take over your entire answer. The best way to introduce the concept of leadership in a "team player" question is to mention it under the heading of flexibility. You would basically say that you are very flexible and take more of a lead when the situation calls for it. To avoid allowing leadership to take over your answer, I would suggest that you only mention it at the end of your answer, as a conclusion.

8.8 Give an example of a recent situation where you played an important role in a team

This question is asking for a recent example. Typically, this means the last few months (though you could probably get away with a one-year-old example).

Also, note the focus of the question is on a situation where teamwork is important as opposed to a situation where you were a good team player. However, you should not be fooled by this; it is a question about you and your ability to demonstrate good team-playing abilities. You must therefore find an example where you played a key role.

Examples that you can use

Identify a situation in your recent past where you have had the opportunity to demonstrate a range of team-playing skills set out in the previous question. This could be a situation where you:

- Participated in the organisation of an event or project such as organising a seminar, regular teaching sessions, health camps, awareness programmes, etc.

- Had to deal with a complex patient, where team playing was important. In order to make the answer interesting you would need to find an example where you had to deal with a multi-disciplinary team, for example. You could then explain how you participated in the debate about the management and ongoing care of the patient, and how you interacted with all members of the team to achieve a safe discharge.

- Had to deal with an emergency by using the staff resources available, whilst maintaining constant communication with your seniors so that they could have an input into the process and would be fully briefed by the time they arrived. Note that, in order to highlight as many skills as possible, you would need to ensure that the situation was complex enough to show how your role was key to the success of the team. For example, if your seniors are there with you and they are managing the situation themselves (e.g. crash call), you are losing the opportunity to emphasise the communication aspect of your role in keeping them up to date.

Example of an ineffective answer

"I work every day as part of a team, dealing with my immediate colleagues, nurses and other doctors. I am aware of my limitations and seek help when necessary, and I communicate well with everyone in the team. I am willing to help and motivate others."

This answer is too vague and general. In fact, it does little more than summarise the job description. Also, it does not actually answer the question, which is asking for an example of a recent situation, i.e. a specific scenario, in which you were involved.

Another example of an ineffective answer

"I had an elderly patient who wanted to self-discharge because she was worried about her dog. I talked to the nurse and the consultant, and eventually the patient agreed to stay one more day. The patient left the hospital the next day and was happy with the way she had been dealt with."

This answer follows the STAR structure (see 5.2), which is a plus point. It starts well by explaining the context that leads to the team action being started. However, the "Action" section contains very little information:

- Why did the candidate talk to the nurse or the consultant? Probably because the consultant is responsible for the patient and had to be informed. As for the nurse, it might have been because she had a good relationship with the patient and a good understanding of their psychological issues too through the rapport she had built with that patient. This needs to be explained.

- Did the candidate do anything else that would have shown him/her to be a good team player? Such as taking the initiative to contact social services or asking the patient if the relatives could be involved? (They can become part of the team too.)

This answer basically needs more detail about what was done and why it was done. In addition, the "Result" section is partially addressing the wrong point. As well as highlighting that the problem was satisfactorily resolved, it should emphasise that this was the result of teamwork.

Example of an effective answer

"Three months ago I was on call, taking admissions from GPs and Accident and Emergency. I was the only Foundation Year 2 doctor on-site, with my Registrar being busy in theatre and my consultant on call from home. A patient presented with <Emergency> which required admission and an emergency operation. Whilst

I was resuscitating the patient, I asked the Foundation Year 1 to call the Registrar in theatre as I felt it was important to inform him as soon as possible. The Registrar informed the FY1 that he would be busy for at least two hours and I therefore took the decision to call the consultant as well, who announced that he would come in and see the patient.

At the same time I asked one of the nurse practitioners to call the anaesthetist and help prepare the theatre so that everything would be ready by the time the consultant arrived. Throughout this time I kept in constant communication with the consultant in order to ensure that he was fully briefed. The patient was taken to theatre within minutes of the consultant's arrival and made a successful post-operative recovery. By coordinating the team at a time that was stressful for all involved (patient and doctors) I helped achieve this result. This taught me how crucial communication is in ensuring that the whole team functions well."

Note the absence of much detailed clinical information (totally irrelevant for the purpose of highlighting team playing), the concise but informative introduction, and the manner in which the main components of team playing are highlighted throughout the example by the candidate, including:

- Recognising your limitations
- Informing his seniors and keeping them up to date about developments
- Informing other colleagues about developments that are relevant to them (the anaesthetist)
- Using other team members to help out, based on their skills level
- Getting things done (stabilising the patient, preparing the theatre, etc.).

Also note how the conclusion keeps the mind of the interviewer focused on the candidate's skills by not only explaining the outcome in a concise manner but also highlighting what he/she did that made it possible to achieve it, and what he learnt from it. Without this element of reflection, the answer would achieve a low score.

8.9	Give an example of a situation where you failed to act as a good team player

Like all negative questions asking you to incriminate yourself, you must make sure that you choose an example which helps you sell your potential. The interviewers will be testing:

- Your self-awareness, i.e. your ability to recognise your faults, reflect on situations and determine what you did wrong.

- Your ability to learn from your bad experiences and change your behaviour accordingly.

Examples that you can discuss

Essentially, you need to consider the qualities of a good team player (see 8.7) and identify whether you have examples of situations where you acted against any of these. This could include a situation where:

- You failed to complete a task that you were entrusted to do and, when you realised that you would struggle to complete it, you did not inform the person who had asked you to do it.

- You did complete the task or project that you were entrusted to run but you were so busy that you did not give it your full attention and the quality of your work suffered, i.e. you became complacent.

- You had some important personal issues to resolve and thought it would be okay to leave a little early. You chose not to let anyone know and, unfortunately, someone actually needed your help.

- You attended a meeting where you had a "heated debate" with someone because you focused a bit too much on trying to impose your point of view rather than listening to what they had to say.

- One of your colleagues was struggling or needed some help but you felt it was someone else's job to do it.

- You were uncomfortable changing your approach to a particular problem despite receiving advice from colleagues because you felt you were right (but ended up being wrong).

- Someone suggested a change in working practices but you resisted the change because you couldn't see the point. You failed to consider the new approach and ended up causing friction.

- You felt that something was not quite right in the way some aspects of patient care or departmental life were organised and decided to let it go because you felt your input would not make much difference (or that you were about to rotate anyway).

- You had information that would make a difference to a particular issue but did not feel confident raising it (though this may be dangerous to mention because the interviewers may feel that you would be reluctant to report a problem colleague, for example).

- You carried out a task by yourself instead of involving other appropriate people because you felt it would be easier or quicker to get on with it. Your colleagues then became upset (once again, consider this option carefully as your interviewers may view you as having a tendency to work beyond your limitations).

Structuring your answer

To give your answer the maximum impact, you must ensure that the emphasis is on the learning points rather than on your bad behaviour. The following approach would be successful in achieving this:

Situation/Task	Describe the situation, your behaviour and the negative impact that it had (e.g. someone became upset). State clearly why you feel you did not demonstrate appropriate team-playing behaviour.
Action	Explain how you resolved the problem at the time (e.g. did you have to work harder to compensate for your failure, or attempt to build bridges with colleagues you had upset?)
Result/Reflect	How did the story finish? What did you learn from the situation and how do you feel it has altered your behaviour. This is the most crucial part of the answer. Make sure that there is a strong learning point and, if you can (and if you've got time), briefly describe another situation which demonstrates that you have now altered your behaviour.

8.10 Do you work better on your own or as part of a team?

This question is often misunderstood and sees candidates rushing to reassure the interviewers that, since they are good team players, they work better as part of a team. The answer is slightly more complex and requires you to demonstrate that, although you are, of course, a good team player, you can also work independently (though still within the remit of a team), i.e. that you are not someone who requires constant support to get on with their work.

One way to structure the answer is to have two sections: one where you describe how you can work independently, followed by a section on how you can also work as part of a team. Alternatively, you can structure your answer around different types of work that you do, showing how you can be independent and also a team player. As usual, you will be expected to back up your claims with examples from your personal practice.

Example of an effective answer

"The answer to this question is that I can work well both as part of a team and independently, depending on what the situation calls for. When I arrive in the morning, I ensure that the list for the ward round is ready on time, with all the investigation results. Although I take full ownership of this task, it is a clearly defined role and often requires me to use my own initiative; by fulfilling this job well, I function as a team player at the same time. Indeed, I need to anticipate what information my colleagues are likely to need when making management decisions; I also often need to liaise with other departments when information is missing, which requires good communication and, sometimes, diplomacy.

When I undertake my audit projects, a lot of the work required consists of data collection and analysis. I like to take full responsibility for all of this and make sure that I deliver what is required by working independently. However, I also involve my senior colleagues when I need to discuss a particular issue relating to the project; and if one of my junior colleagues is keen to get involved, I will make sure that they can take part in the project too.

I think that part of being a good team player is also to be able to undertake roles and work independently, delivering what the team requires of you, whilst ensuring that you maintain constant communication. I feel that it is something that I am particularly good at and my colleagues' feedback is that I am a very proactive and entrepreneurial individual who is, at the same time, very attentive to others' needs and also a very good communicator."

8.11 What makes you a good leader?

What is leadership?

Leadership can be described in three words: – **C**hange – **P**eople – **R**esults

---

Initiating and implementing Change
A leader is someone who has a vision of how departments or teams should develop or change and is able to drive that change. He/she is able to question conventional wisdom and current practice, to encourage others to develop their own ideas and to implement new protocols, guidelines or new ways of working. This involves building relationships with others, not just within your own environment but also with others outside, to ensure greater collaboration and achieve common goals. Leadership is also about identifying and understanding the impact of internal and external politics and acting accordingly. That involves negotiating and influencing others, building consensus and gaining cooperation from others to ensure that the right information is obtained and that common objectives are achieved.

Developing People (and creating a positive environment)
A leader takes people with him/her towards the objectives that he/she has set and makes sure that he/she creates an environment in which people can develop, work together and cooperate, and where there are good mechanisms in place to resolve conflicts constructively.

Delivering Results
This is the ability to meet set goals and expectations. This includes an ability to make decisions that lead to tangible results by applying knowledge, analysing problems, and calculating risks. Delivering results is the aspect of leadership to which you are most usually exposed as a trainee, and the closest to management. Essentially, it is about organising a team, planning and delegating, and getting things done.

You don't have to be a clinical director to be a leader!

Leadership is a real skill that anyone can demonstrate. You don't have to be a consultant or a chief executive to exercise leadership. I am often struck by the number of people who ask me at my courses: "How do they expect us to demonstrate leadership when we are only trainees?" In truth, you probably started demonstrating leadership very early in your career and even before. For example, anyone who has had to deal with a busy on-call or with multiple emergencies on their own or with limited resources would be demonstrating leadership – even leading a ward round and the organisation surrounding that may be an example.

This section should help you clarify your thoughts and will prompt you to think about your own examples.

Qualities of a leader

From the description of leadership set out above, you can see that, in order to be a good leader, you will need to exhibit the following qualities:

Approachable	Encouraging	Integrity
Assertive	Fair	Open-minded
Clear communicator	Fast learner	Organised
Consistent	Flexible	Patient
Constructive	Good listener	Resilient
Creative	Honest	Supportive
Decisive	Innovative	Tenacious
Diplomatic		

Answering the question

What makes you a good leader will be a mixture of the responsibilities that you take and your personal qualities, both of which you can derive from the issues above. Leadership is a vast topic and you should ensure that you focus on three or four areas or skills that you feel represent you and your experience best; attempting to discuss everything will either result in a very superficial or a very long answer.

Example of an effective answer

"One of my strengths as a leader is that I take ownership of a task, a project or a problem when it is given to me. I also involve the other members of my team to ensure that we work well together towards completing that project. For example, during on-calls I may have several complicated cases to deal with at once; at times the Registrar and consultant may not be immediately available either because they are busy somewhere else, or because they are on call from home. In such a situation, I aim to make decisions about how we should prioritise the patients, which member of the team would be best placed to handle each patient, whether we can deal with the issues by ourselves and how likely we are to require assistance from senior colleagues. As a leader in these stressful situations, I feel that I am very good at keeping the team together by maintaining good communication with everyone, by making myself available if colleagues have queries or questions they want to discuss and also by making decisions when they need to be made. Sometimes this may require seeking advice from someone more senior or more experienced.

As a leader, I am also very supportive and encouraging towards my colleagues, trying my absolute best to encourage my juniors to consolidate their skills and experience, and to develop new ones. For example, when I do an audit, I make a point of involving junior colleagues in collecting and analysing the data. As I review patients in the morning, I also make sure that I identify interesting cases that we could review as a team in order to consolidate our knowledge. I often use these in monthly workshops that I organise for those taking the membership exams and also encourage junior trainees to present these cases at departmental teaching sessions. I have found these activities particularly effective for developing a good relationship between all team members and making everyone feel involved.

Finally, I have a good ability to engage with people, even when conflicts develop. For example, I have had to deal with GPs who insisted that a patient with seemingly little wrong with them should be admitted, with a nurse who refused to administer a drug which she felt contravened hospital policy, with relatives who were adamant that the patient was not being treated well or even with a Registrar who made decisions I believed were not in the best interests of patients. In these situations, I have always been very good at keeping calm (and in fact this is one of the comments that often comes back in my feedback forms) and at trying to find a constructive way of resolving the problem."

This answer is effective because:

- It has three points which are clearly signposted at the start of each paragraph and demonstrate wide-ranging experience, with examples.

- Each point is expanded just enough to show the extent of the candidate's experience.

- The candidate reflects on his skills by demonstrating their impact on others. Bringing feedback into the answer (last paragraph) helps to introduce some objectivity into the answer

- The candidate uses a positive language and also appears realistic by presenting the image of someone who, despite being confident, can also involve others and ask for assistance.

8.12 Give an example of a situation where you showed leadership

Choosing the best example

For this question, you should familiarise yourself with the role and qualities of a leader discussed in the previous questions and try to determine which examples would enable you to best present your leadership abilities.

Initiating and implementing change
- Any situation where you identified a problem in the workplace and took the initiative to implement a solution. Maybe you spotted some inefficiency or lack of compliance, did an audit to identify the extent of the problem and then tried to encourage your team to change its practice. Perhaps you identified some training issues and took it upon yourself to liaise with other key team members to change some aspects of training

- Situations where you held positions of responsibility and were instrumental in making decisions that impacted on other people (for example, if you were on the board of some student committee at medical school).

Developing people and creating a positive environment
- Any team environment/meeting where you have encouraged and managed differences of opinions (e.g. ward round, MDT meetings)

- Situations where you have dealt with a conflict with colleagues in a constructive manner (e.g. underperforming colleague)

- Projects or tasks where you played a key role in encouraging and supporting juniors or other colleagues, developing their skills and abilities by providing feedback and encouragement, and providing them with opportunities to become involved in interesting or stretching projects (e.g. audit, teaching or other projects)

- Situations where you sought to encourage a positive team spirit. This could be either through encouragement whilst dealing with a difficult work situation, or even outside of work (e.g. by organising team events such as quizzes, sport tournaments, etc.).

Delivering results
- Competently managing a difficult case with little senior help
- Dealing with multiple emergencies in an under-resourced environment
- Dealing with a difficult patient or a complaint
- Being confronted with a sensitive problem with no immediate help (e.g. child protection issue or any other challenging situation)

- Facing tight deadlines to complete a complex project (e.g. publication for which you need advice from a senior who couldn't care less)
- Negotiating admission of a patient onto a ward where the ward doctor on-call refused
- Negotiating admission of a patient to ITU where the ITU doctor was reluctant to agree
- Requesting a scan from Radiology, who refused to perform it
- Situation where a GP or another doctor requested something unreasonable and you needed to "educate" him about your position
- Any negotiating situation outside of medicine, for example if you were in charge of organising an event, or part of a committee, and had to influence other people to help you with your project, when they were reluctant to engage.

Delivering the answer

Delivering the answer should be done using the STAR approach (see 5.2), ensuring that you use the story as a backdrop to your leadership skills (the whole point of the question is to give you an opportunity to show off your leadership skills, and not just the story itself).

Example of an effective answer	
Situation/Task	"A few months ago, a child was admitted onto the paediatric HDU ward feeling unwell with diabetic ketoacidosis. During the night, the child's condition deteriorated.
Action	Since the change was significant and unexpected I informed the consultant so that he could advise then and, should I need his help later on, he would be aware of the situation. At the same time, I also informed the anaesthetist and asked for his assessment in case the child required ITU admission later.
	I started to manage the child accordingly, using an established protocol, and he gradually showed signs of improvement. I therefore decided it was safe to keep the child on the HDU and organised for nurses to check the child at 30-minute intervals and let me know of any changes in his condition. This enabled me to provide care to other patients whilst keeping up to date with the child's development. I also explained that I would return to review him once I had checked on other patients.
	In the meantime, I met up with the boy's parents in order to keep them updated on their son's situation; this provided them with information, a chance to ask questions and some reassurance. I also arranged for a nurse to check regularly on them to make

	sure they remained happy with developments. Throughout the process I kept my consultant involved where necessary; this meant he had a clear picture of events and would be able to answer any questions from parents later. As the child's condition improved further, he was transferred to the general paediatrics ward, at which point I involved a diabetic nurse and a dietician who talked to the child and the parents about insulin and the importance of diet.
Result	When the consultant arrived, the parents were keen to discuss their son's care with him. With the advance information I had provided for him, he was able to see the parents very quickly after reviewing the child and his notes. This proved very reassuring for the parents; they also told him that they had been really impressed with the care I had given to their son and the explanation they'd received from me.
Reflect	This was a medical emergency. I placed the patient's care and treatment as the highest priority, I was working with a good team and with good planning, delegation and appropriate communication everyone understood their role and completed it well. By carefully coordinating the actions of a wide range of colleagues, I was able to make sure the team delivered efficient and safe care to the patient and his family."

This example is effective because it describes in detail the candidate's actions, with sufficient but not excessive clinical information, and clear reflection at the end of the answer.

8.13 What is the difference between management and leadership?

In a nutshell, leadership is setting a new direction or vision for a group and developing colleagues in a team. Management is about controlling or directing people/resources in a group according to principles or values that have already been established.

The difference between leadership and management can be illustrated by considering what happens when you have one without the other.

Leadership without management ... sets a direction or vision that others follow, without considering too much how the new direction is going to be achieved. Other people then have to work hard in the trail that is left behind, picking up the pieces and making it work. In medicine, this could be a consultant who asks junior doctors or nurses to manage a patient in a certain way without making sure that it is realistic or without understanding the hurdles that could be met on the way.

Management without leadership ... controls resources to maintain the status quo or ensure things happen according to already-established plans. For example, a referee manages a sports game, but does not usually provide "leadership" because there is no new change, no new direction – the referee is controlling resources to ensure that the laws of the game are followed and status quo is maintained. In medicine, this would be a doctor who ensures that protocols and guidelines are followed without questioning, when necessary, whether they are actually applicable or relevant. It would also be a doctor who gets things done but does not worry about finding opportunities to train and develop his juniors.

Leadership combined with management ... does both – it sets a new direction *and* manages the resources to achieve it, for example a newly elected prime minister.

8.14 Give an example of a situation where a new and different approach to a patient of yours proved beneficial

What is this question about?

Essentially the question is asking you to describe a situation where your first approach was unsuccessful and where you then changed your strategy of approach to achieve your objective. This could include situations where:

- A patient was reluctant to go ahead with one of your recommendations and where you had to take a different approach in your communication to ensure that they got the message.

- A patient with whom you used a first approach that revealed some hidden issues, which then prompted you to choose a different approach. For example, you may have adopted a "standard" approach to the problem but then gained information from the patient that indicated there were deeper psychological issues at stake that needed to be resolved as part of the same process.

This question is testing three skills:

- Your ability to think laterally about a difficult situation, using your knowledge of the patient/situation and the resources available to you in order to find a solution that will drive you towards a successful outcome. (Note that this could include involving other people such as relatives, other doctors, etc. in which case you may be able to include an element of teamwork in your answer.)

- Your communication skills in relation to the patient.

- The manner in which you are able to build and maintain a rapport with the patient to achieve your desired objective, whilst not compromising your integrity but preserving respect for the patient's values and choices.

Delivering the answer

This is a question asking for a specific example so you should use the STAR structure (see 5.2), ensuring that you do not provide too much clinical information, that you describe clearly the steps that you took to achieve the desired result and that you mention the outcome. If appropriate, you should reflect on the situation to highlight what you did well.

Example of an ineffective answer

"An obese 42-year-old HGV driver came to my clinic with a high blood sugar level. His GP had referred him to the diabetic clinic twice (he had Type 2 diabetes) and, each time, the patient had failed to attend. Despite my best efforts to explain the situation to the patient and encourage him to attend, he was not listening attentively and was being uncooperative. I felt a stronger approach would be required to spur the patient into action. I told him that, unless he was admitted into hospital and treated, there would be long-term complications to his diabetes, such as loss of eyesight, nerve damage, heart disease and stroke."

The above answer has many good points: it deals with a specific example, the situation is fairly clear and the clinical information is reduced to the bare minimum. However, it seems a little harsh. The candidate is saying "He wouldn't listen so I scared him to make him comply". This needs to be softened. In particular, he should spend more time demonstrating how he approached the patient in the first place in order to demonstrate why the second approach was then necessary.

Also the candidate has missed out the "Result" part of the answer. This makes it look very odd and even scary to a point. You simply don't feel that there was a rapport between the patient and the doctor, or any attempt by the doctor to try his very best before escalating his approach. The answer should therefore focus more around the communication aspect and how the doctor interacted with the patient, rather than just about what the doctor felt and what he said.

Example of an effective answer

Situation/Task	"An obese 42-year-old HGV driver came to my clinic with a high blood sugar level and a urinary tract infection. His history revealed that his GP had referred him to the diabetic clinic twice for Type 2 diabetes and that the patient had failed to attend both appointments. On enquiring about the reasons for his non-attendance, the patient mentioned that he was scared of being prescribed insulin as it would lead to the loss of his HGV licence.
Action	My first approach to the patient's reaction was to listen to him carefully and then explain that I understood his dilemma, emphasising the solutions we could find. I took him through the features of Type 2 diabetes and explained that there were ways in which it could be controlled. In view of his worries, I reassured him that insulin would probably not be necessary at this stage. I sensed that the patient was not listening attentively and was being uncooperative. As he had already missed two appointments and was showing few signs of engaging with my proposed plan, I felt that a stronger approach was re-

	quired to encourage him to listen and take appropriate action. After discussing my proposed approach with my Registrar, I explained to the patient that, unless he was admitted into hospital and treated, there would be long-term complications to his diabetes, such as loss of eyesight, nerve damage, heart disease and stroke.
Result/Reflect	This resulted in a drastic change in the patient's attitude and he very quickly agreed to our management plan. A few months later, the patient thanked me for my empathic but assertive approach as he felt I had saved his life."

This answer is more balanced: showing empathy, discussing with the Registrar and then adapting the style of communication to the situation and the patient's reaction.

It would be easy to mishandle the question by taking a very clinical perspective; this would lead you straight to disaster. There is no harm in presenting clinical information as was done above, but only to the extent that it helps towards the story. In the example above, it was necessary to demonstrate the gravity of the patient's condition and the extent to which the patient was "scared" into concordance.

Finally, beware of words that may sound harsher than you mean them to be. For example, "I told" is very direct whilst "I explained" is softer.

8.15	Describe a time when you were unsure whether what you were being told represented the patient's true thoughts or feelings

What type of examples can you discuss?

The question does not tell you whether it is the patient who is not telling you their true thoughts, or whether it is a relative who is telling you something that does not match the patient's thoughts or feelings.

If it is the patient, then it may be because they are frightened of what will happen to them if they reveal their thoughts or feelings. This may be a patient who is scared about their own health problems or diagnosis, a patient who hides part of their history to avoid confronting the reality of their illness, or an elderly patient who is keen to have their health problems resolved but is not keen to be taken into care. They might also be worried about becoming a burden on their relatives.

If it is a relative, it may be that they are trying to forcibly influence the patient into a position that suits them rather than the patient. More often it is relatives who feel they have little or no control over their family's healthcare. They often want to help and, whilst the strong expression of their views may be well intentioned, it is often misplaced or misguided.

Which skills are being tested?

The interviewers will be testing:

- Your listening skills, with a particular interest in how you recognised that there was a problem – recognising the issue will come from your own judgement of the situation based maybe on inconsistencies in the story that you are getting from the patient, their body language, the way they express themselves (for example, by being vague), etc. Ultimately this will come from your ability to listen to the patient.

- Your empathy, sensitivity and diplomacy. Dealing with the issue is complex and requires you to gain the patient's confidence in order to put them back on the right track. This requires diplomacy and sensitivity.

- Teamwork. You may need to involve:
    - a nurse – they often have a more in-depth relationship with the patients simply because they may be more empathic than doctors and have more time to spend with patients.
    - the GP – if there is time to make decisions and the patient can be helped through counselling or simply by having an opportunity to discuss issues.
    - the relatives, if needed. They may be crucial in reassuring the patient.
    - your seniors.

If you judge that the relatives are causing the problem (for example, by forcing the patient to adopt a particular attitude against his/her will) you may have to use other tools to minimise their possible negative influence on the patient. This could include involving seniors, behaving in an assertive but sensitive manner, spending time with the relatives (after all, there may be a valid reason or fear behind their behaviour), etc.

Example of an ineffective answer

"One of my patients wanted to self-discharge because she felt her dog would be in danger if she did not get back home as soon as possible. I suggested that she called a relative so that they could look after the animal but she was adamant that she needed to do it herself. This prompted me to think that there was more to her story and, after much discussion, I concluded that she was worried about the anaesthesia. In order to resolve the situation I arranged for the patient to have a second discussion with the anaesthetist and also arranged for a nurse to sit in with her. After the discussion the patient was happy and went through with the operation."

This answer is not "bad". It has a number of positive aspects:
- It deals with a specific situation.
- The introduction is descriptive and effective in setting out the situation.
- It addresses the right type of issue.

On the negative side, it describes what the doctor did, but not really why he/she thought or acted like this. In other words, the answer needs more depth and needs to highlight how the doctor used his/her skills to resolve the situation.

Look at the following statement: "This prompted me to think that there was more to her story and, after much discussion, I concluded that she was worried about the anaesthesia." Essentially, it looks as if the doctor has jumped to a conclusion without really explaining how it came about. The whole process has been summarised by "after much discussion". The candidate would need to go into more detail about that conversation and discuss how they spent time with the patient, discussing the situation and their fears, eventually picking up on parts of the conversation that seemed to indicate that she was afraid of having an anaesthetic.

The candidate also needs to emphasise how they used listening skills and empathy to gain the patient's trust and confidence. Perhaps they also asked a nurse to have a conversation with the patient instead because they felt the nurse had a better rapport with the patient and that the patient would open up more to them.

Example of an effective answer

Situation/Task	"One of my patients wanted to self-discharge because she felt that her dog would be in danger if she did not get back home as soon as possible. I suggested that she called a relative so that they could look after the animal but she was adamant that she needed to do it herself. This prompted me to think that there was more to her story and that, maybe, she feared the operation she was due to have the next day.
Action	During a quiet period, I asked a nurse to make sure that I would not be disturbed. I sat down with the patient and asked her gently to tell me about her dog. I listened patiently to her, showing an interest in her story and occasionally asking questions. As the patient opened up to me, I felt more comfortable introducing the subject of her own health and the operation. I could feel that she wanted to express her fears but that she was reluctant to admit to the problem, perhaps because she did not want to appear foolish. I gently explained what the operation entailed and reassured her about the anaesthesia. In order to avoid giving the patient the impression that I was pressurising her, I asked the nurse to spend some time with her. To reassure the patient further, I arranged a meeting with the anaesthetist and arranged for the relatives to discuss the care of the dogs with the patient.
Result	After a few hours of concerted teamwork and sensitive communication, the patient agreed to remain in hospital and the surgery went ahead as scheduled, with a successful outcome. I feel that I played an important role in achieving a good outcome for the patient despite her initial reluctance to open up, not only by recognising some of her unspoken needs but also by giving her the time and attention that she needed to open up, without coercing her."

This example combines teamwork and communication skills in a relatively detailed manner. To have an impact, you must make sure that your answers are as personal as they can be by drawing on the relevant detail of the experience that you have accumulated over the years. The above example also shows you how you can transform an "okay" answer into a much more precise answer simply by expanding on one or two ideas that you raised, highlighting how you used your skills in practice to achieve the desired result.

8.16	Describe a situation when you had to use creative thinking to solve a problem at work

What is creative thinking?

Many candidates who are confronted with this question struggle to find appropriate examples, not because they are short of experience but simply because they struggle with the wording of the question, and particularly the meaning of the term "creative thinking". If you struggle with some words in the question, it is of course perfectly acceptable to ask the interviewers for clarification so that you have a chance to present the best possible answer, though of course it may cost you a small amount of marks. However, losing a few marks for seeking clarification is far better than scoring none for going down completely the wrong path.

"Creative thinking" refers to the fact that you have used your imagination and initiative to resolve a problem. In the marking schedule, the interviewers would be looking for the following indicators:

- Capacity to use logic and lateral thinking to solve problems and make decisions
- Capacity to think beyond the obvious, with an analytical and flexible mind
- Capacity to bring a range of approaches to problem solving
- Demonstrates effective judgement and decision-making skills.

Examples you can discuss

The question relates to a situation with which you were unfamiliar and for which you had to use your brain power to develop a sensible and effective solution. This may include situations where:

- You had to deal with a patient who presented with a condition that you were unfamiliar with.

- Your senior asked you to organise something that you had never organised before (educational meeting, audit project, rota, etc.).
- You had to deal with several tasks at the same time, which looked completely impossible to you at the time (for example, routine work and several emergencies all at the same time).

- You have a patient who looks like he has a particular condition but something tells you that there is more to it than meets the eye. Your creative thinking leads you to do some reading in text books and on the Internet, before having a chat with your Registrar. You also feel that another doctor from another ward can help, so you contact them and arrange a discussion on the patient's condition to find a solution to your problem.

- You work in a hospital where the rota is imposing too many constraints on junior doctors (perhaps they have made a mess of implementing the European Working Time Directive). You come up with a solution of your own, discuss it with your colleagues and then arrange a meeting with a consultant to discuss the problems caused by the current system and to offer your own ideas. As a result, your proposal is implemented.

- You are running a clinic where you constantly have the same problem with patients. For example, there is some simple information that they need to take away with them after the clinic but that information often gets scribbled on a piece of paper, which they lose. You take the initiative to produce a pro forma slip, which doctors can complete quickly by ticking the right boxes and which patients are less likely to ignore.

- You have discovered that members of your team often forget to consider certain points in their history taking, which slows down patient management and may lead to errors. You know that the current system has been implemented by a consultant who thinks that it works well, and you need to convince everyone that the system needs to be changed. Your creative thinking leads you to use diplomacy and tact to highlight the issue and to offer a counter-solution without upsetting the consultant in question.

- You are on call, facing a difficult case, and none of your seniors are available for help. You can then describe the research you did to find a solution and how you used other resources available (nurses' advice, other juniors/seniors from other wards) to solve your problem.

Delivering the answer

As this is a question asking for an example, you will need to use the STAR approach used in such previous questions (see 5.2). You should conclude on a personal note, for example, by mentioning how the situation helped you gain confidence in your own abilities to handle complex scenarios or how it made you realise how important it was to use the resources available to you and to work as a team.

Example of an effective answer

Situation/Task   "In my hospital, the mess room is located outside the main hospital and, as a result, very few doctors use it. This makes it very difficult for doctors to take appropriate breaks as they are forced to stay within the clinical area and therefore any breaks are regularly interrupted. It also makes handing over a difficult exercise as there is no quiet area in which it can be done effectively. As a result, a number of doctors have chosen to hand over through written notes whilst others simply may not hand over properly.

Action	I suggested to my consultant that we should consider having the mess room within the confines of the main hospital building so that it encourages doctors to use it both for personal and professional purposes. In order to convince my consultant without using up too much of his time, I prepared a single A4 sheet of paper highlighting the issues associated with the situation and explaining the benefits of implementing the change. I explained that patient care would be improved by opening a mess room within the hospital. As well as enabling doctors to have proper breaks, it would facilitate contact between colleagues from the same and different departments and could be used to have systematic handover meetings in a quiet setting. I also set out a number of measures to make the room attractive to all doctors and encourage usage, such as installing a coffee machine.
Result/Reflect	My suggestion was subsequently approved by management on the advice of my consultant and is currently being implemented. This was an issue that had often been talked about amongst my colleagues but never addressed. Most people felt that it would be too much hard work to convince anyone to effect a change, particularly since all the consultants never seemed to have any time to discuss such matters. However, by anticipating the information that they would need to make a decision, gathering all the information and presenting a case in a simple and concise format, I was able to help management reach a quick and unanimous decision, which benefited the whole team."

This answer is effective because the issue is clearly set out and well explained. The "Action" section is not confined to what the doctor did, but explains why he/she took such steps and demonstrates that the doctor anticipates the impact of his/her actions on others. This reflects a good level of influencing skills (i.e. the ability to get things done without coercing anyone), which would score highly.

The example above is not a clinical example; however, it would be perfectly acceptable to discuss a clinical scenario, using the same principles. If you have any doubt as to whether the interviewers require a clinical scenario or not, ask them to clarify the wording of the question.

8.17 Tell us about a mistake that you have made

What the question is testing

This question is testing your ability to recognise that you make mistakes, to take responsibility for your mistakes, to sort them out, to reflect on your experience, modify your behaviour accordingly and ensure that others benefit from your experience too.

Many candidates are reluctant to discuss their mistakes because they feel that it will present them as bad doctors. However, with this question, the interviewers are trying to establish that you are safe in a realistic context; as far as you are concerned, this means demonstrating that, when mistakes happen, you can deal with them appropriately (and not that you never make mistakes. If you said that, you would score zero).

Structuring an answer

You will need to follow the STAR structure (see 5.2). For this question, this will mean bringing the following items into your answer, all of which would be reflected in the marking scheme:

Situation/Task	Describe the scenario (keeping the clinical information to the strict minimum necessary to the comprehension of the story). Explain what the mistake was and its impact (i.e. how did that affect the patient, if at all).
Action	Explain the clinical steps that you followed to resolve the problem and make sure that the patient was safe. Describe which other members of the team you involved and why you needed to involve them. Describe how you communicated with the patient or relatives about the mistake made (this is often neglected by most candidates, thus costing them valuable marks).
Result/Reflect	Reflect on the scenario and explain what you have learnt from it. Explain how it changed your practice, perhaps giving a quick example of a different situation where you acted differently. Explain how you ensured that others learnt from it (for example, by raising the problem at a team meeting/ sending an email to others). If you completed a critical incident form, don't forget to mention it.

Which mistakes can you mention?

A good answer will discuss a mistake which is:

- Personal, i.e. your mistake and not that of another colleague. If you talk about someone else's mistake you will miss the opportunity to demonstrate your own integrity.

- Interesting, i.e. which has some element of drama. If the mistake is boring to describe, it is likely to score low. Similarly, if you choose a mistake that is fairly common then you are less likely to impress, unless the consequences were significant enough to make the whole answer interesting.

- Safe. You don't want to appear completely incompetent. Safe does not mean that no harm was caused to the patient, but that if there was harm or risk of serious harm you identified it quickly and took immediate steps to resolve the problem. You do want to avoid discussing a mistake where the patient died, though. Answers of the type "The patient died but I learnt a lot" never sound that impressive. Examples which are safe would include any near misses, any situation where the patient was inconvenienced or non-emergency care was delayed, or even any situation where the patient was placed at risk but you recognised it before much harm could be caused. Everyone on your panel will know what being a junior doctor is like. There is no point pretending that you are perfect.

- Good learning ground. Half the marks will relate to the learning points that you drew from the experience and how you changed your practice. If your example is too safe, you are unlikely to have any interesting learning points and will end up scoring a low mark. For this reason you want to avoid any mistakes which are not yours, any mistakes which are caused by a system failure and, for surgeons, any mistakes which are in fact recognised complications since it is only with hindsight that you could say that something could have been done differently.

Here are a few examples of mistakes that could be used. For all clinical mistakes it is important to include the fact that you completed an incident form. If you did not, be prepared to justify this – you may have to admit that the failure to do so was an oversight and a learning point in its own right. This should help you think about your own experience and formulate your own answer:

- Flushing a venflon with lidnocaine instead of saline because the label looked similar and since you were in a hurry you did not take the time to double-check. You would explain how you managed the patient clinically after the mistake was made (moved to resus, cardiac monitoring, called for help from your Registrar, anticipating potential complications and ensuring that all bases were covered). You would then raise the issue of patient communication including reassuring him/her, explaining how you plan to deal with the consequences, apologising and mentioning how you plan to ensure that the same mistake won't happen again. You can then discuss how you changed practice as a result (e.g. this taught you the importance of double-checking your actions) and how this led to a change in the labelling system.

- Giving a patient a dose of antibiotics, not realising that they were allergic. This could have happened because you made the assumption that they were not allergic (the drug chart did not say so, or you just did not remember to check) or perhaps because the bracelet indicating they were allergic was hidden by a bandage. In your answer, you would explain how you kept an eye on the patient to ensure that they did not develop any problems. Hopefully, the patient did not react in this particular case; otherwise you will need to explain which steps you took to treat the clinical problem. Explain that you called for help and communicated with the patient appropriately (explaining, reassuring, apologising). Finally, reflect on the reason why you made the mistake and how you have since changed your practice.

- Discharging a patient with inappropriate medication. You may have spotted the mistake yourself and recalled the patient, or the mistake may have been spotted because the patient turned up a few days later with a more severe problem.

- Failing to plan for a potential complication prior to performing a procedure, as a result of which you were not prepared when it did happen. You then had to call for help to resolve the problem. For this mistake to be effective, you will need to discuss a complication that you should have planned for but somehow didn't. If no one ever plans for it because it is rare then it isn't really a mistake.

- Failing to take into account a patient's co-morbidities (perhaps you were in a hurry, or the notes were so thick that you made assumptions).

The above mistakes are all of a clinical nature. There are other mistakes you can discuss, which are of a managerial or communication nature. These include:

- Delegating a task to a colleague (e.g. junior doctor, nurse) assuming that they would know what to do and how to do it. They didn't and, as a result, patient care was delayed and/or confusion ensued.

- Communicating important information to a patient assuming they would understand it, when in fact they did not. As a result, they did not comply with your instructions. This could be because you were falsely reassured by their behaviour towards you or because you forgot to check their understanding.

- Being a bit too direct with a patient, not realising that in fact they were very sensitive. As a result, you risked causing them more distress than intended or compromising their trust in you.

At an interview, you can mention any mistake, unless the interviewers have directed you towards one particular type. For example, if simply asked for "a mistake", you could mention a clinical or non-clinical mistake. If asked specifically for a clinical mistake, then you would need to find a clinical scenario; fobbing off the interviewers by presenting a non-clinical scenario would result in a low mark. If in doubt, ask them.

Some interviewers will ask for a *recent* example. This usually means the last 6 to 12 months.

Playing safe v taking risks

Having viewed the feedback received by hundreds of candidates over dozens of specialties, I can comfortably say that those who score the highest on this question are candidates who present mistakes where they were actively involved and from which they will have learnt a lot from a personal point of view.

Before the interview, you must decide whether you wish to play safe by presenting an average mistake or a non-clinical mistake, thereby guaranteeing yourself half the marks; or whether you want to be more daring by presenting a more dramatic mistake, which, although risky, may yield you much higher marks if you can explain it properly using the steps highlighted earlier.

8.18 Describe a situation when you demonstrated professional integrity as a doctor

Many candidates have little understanding of the word "integrity", which then leads to poorly positioned answers. Integrity is a crucial part of the GMC's *Good Medical Practice* and you should therefore show a good understanding not only of the concept but also of how it impacts on your work on a daily basis.

Integrity in your day-to-day work

Integrity refers to your ability to do the right thing when it may be tempting to react unethically for the sake of an easier life. This may be:

- Situations where you have made a mistake, where you would be expected to own up to it and take corrective action (see previous question).

- Situations where you should know how to handle a particular issue but somehow you don't. Integrity is about admitting your lack of knowledge and working towards addressing it (a lack of integrity would be pretending that you know what to do, which may put your patients and colleagues at risk).

- Situations where you discover that something is wrong and where you take proactive steps to address the situation (for example, if you discover that one of your colleagues has made a mistake, is an alcoholic, takes drugs, has abused a patient or is underperforming/incompetent).

- Situations where you were pressurised to do something that you knew or felt was wrong and where you resisted the pressure (e.g. a relative, a friend or a colleague encouraging you to breach patient confidentiality or a patient wanting you to prescribe a treatment that you know would not work).

- A colleague who wanted a favour that would place you in a difficult position (covering up for a mistake they made, prescribing them controlled drugs, etc.).

Example of an effective answer (using the STAR approach)

Situation/Task   "In my Foundation Year attachment in General Practice, a mother came in with her child, who had a cough, fever and sore throat. The mother insisted that her baby had a chest infection and demanded antibiotics. After a thorough examination of the child, the chest was clear and I diagnosed viral upper respiratory tract infection. In the short term, the child only really needed paracetamol, rehydration and steam inhalation.

The mother became slightly irritated at the fact that I did not wish to consider antibiotics and after having spent some time explaining to her in simple terms why antibiotics would not work in this situation, she did not show any sign of changing her position. She indicated very strongly that she felt I had not been trained properly and that any good doctor would give her the antibiotics she was requesting. She demanded to see my consultant.

Action

The mother was placing me under a lot of pressure to give her what she wanted by attempting to intimidate me. It was important that I kept my cool and did not give in simply to get rid of the problem that I was facing. I provided the mother with a couple of leaflets regarding sore throat and cough from the PRODIGY guideline and told her that I would refer the issue to my consultant for advice straight away.

My consultant explained that the best way forward would be to offer the mother a back-up antibiotic prescription and ask her to come back for it if her child did not improve after two days. I explained to the mother that I would compromise by getting her to follow my advice whilst the back-up prescription, in line with her wishes, would give her the reassurance of antibiotic back-up.

Result/Reflect

The mother left happy and came back to thank me after the child got better without the need for antibiotics. In this situation I maintained my integrity by remaining professional in my relationship with the patient despite the pressure that she was placing on me, by not giving in to a request that I deemed against the best interest of the patient. It also helped to dissipate her anxiety and maintain my credibility by involving a senior colleague appropriately. This example also illustrates the importance of communication in dealing with potential conflicts. In this case, by remaining civil, I avoided a potential complaint."

The STAR approach (see 5.2) provides a clear structure for the story. Each step is properly explained from the candidate's point of view and there is a good level of reflection at the end. The example also clearly shows the candidate as someone who took responsibility for sorting the problem out, highlighting, where appropriate, how professional integrity was maintained.

8.19 What are the advantages and disadvantages of admitting when mistakes are made?

This question not only tests your integrity, but also your understanding of why integrity matters. The question looks very theoretical, calling for a list that you could simply learn and regurgitate; however, obviously, many candidates will come up with a similar list and you therefore need to set yourself apart from the rest by bringing your personal experiences into your answer.

Advantages of admitting when mistakes are made

- You are able to repair the mistake much more quickly because you can involve others in the process.

- You can openly identify areas of possible improvement and gain support from your superiors to deal with them.

- You may originally annoy people but they would be grateful for your honesty. In the long term, owning up to your mistakes may encourage people to trust you more because they know that you are honest.

- If you cover up a mistake for a long time and it is then discovered, the patient may lose trust in you and in the medical profession as a whole. You may be sued or struck off. If you admit the mistake and apologise early enough, the matter is much more likely to be resolved without such drastic consequences.

Disadvantages of admitting when mistakes are made

- Your colleagues and patients may lower their opinion of you.
- You may be sacked, sued, struck off, or all of the aforementioned.
- Patients may lose trust towards you and/or the medical profession.

Bringing examples into your answer

As mentioned earlier, it is crucial that you mention examples in order to make your answer more personal and more interesting; otherwise it will resemble everyone else's answer. When you give examples, keep your descriptions to two or three sentences. Here are a few effective examples:

"...One of the advantages of admitting that you have made a mistake is that you can avoid complaints or at least minimise their impact. For example, I once examined a patient in A&E and prescribed antacid, believing that the patient had indigestion. Later on he was admitted for acute anterior MI. His son was angry. I spent some time discussing the situation with him, and apologised profusely for my mistake. The son accepted my apology gratefully, thanked me for my honesty and left it at that ..."

"...Admitting to a mistake is helpful in maintaining a good relationship with patients providing the communication with the patient is well handled. At the same time, it also helps in gaining support from your superiors to acquire new skills. I was once asked to perform a cervical smear test. Unfortunately, I applied a little too much force as I rotated the spatula. On smearing the sample onto a slide, it contained a little blood. I immediately explained to the patient what had happened and apologised for any pain and inconvenience. She was very understanding and agreed to visit in three months for another smear test. I reported the incident to my senior, who suggested that I undertake further training in the test. Three months later, I successfully performed the procedure on the same patient ..."

"...A possible disadvantage of owning up to your mistakes is that the patient may lose trust in you as a doctor when they learn the truth. I remember a particular example of a situation where I had misplaced a blood sample for a patient and had to take a second one to replace it. Because it was something that was very simple and harmless, I hadn't felt it necessary to tell the patient about the mistake. The patient later came to know about it from a nurse who, as a gesture of goodwill, had asked the patient if she felt okay about the problem. Luckily the patient was very understanding and let the matter go, but I could sense that I had bruised our relationship slightly as a result of my lack of attention to detail. I have worked hard to ensure this does not happen again."

To have an effective answer, all you need is three or four points with a couple of good examples. There is no need to give an example for every single point that you make; illustrating a couple of your points would be sufficient to provide a good balance. Don't be afraid of examples referring to negative consequences, but make sure they illustrate the point without presenting you as useless at your job (see the last example above).

8.20 How do you organise your workload?

At first glance, the question seems straightforward. However, like all questions relating to a generic topic, there is a risk that everyone ends up giving the same answer and therefore you should personalise it by giving suitable examples from your experience in order to stand out, even if the question does not explicitly ask for examples.

Organising your workload

Before you can answer the question effectively, you must identify the different ways in which you organise yourself at work. Don't try to be theoretical and sec-ond-guess a list of ways in which one might organise oneself. Simply think about what you do every day at work (it will make it easier to find suitable examples when you deliver the answer).

Here are a few examples that may be relevant to your situation and which you could describe:

- Making lists of patients and a list of tasks, whether patient related or not. Prioritising your tasks.

- Identifying whether you might require assistance from other people and ensuring they are briefed early enough (and available!).

- Reviewing your list on a regular basis, updating patient details and reprioritising if necessary.

- Delegating tasks to the appropriate colleague/sharing the workload.

- Working efficiently by initiating investigations you need to do as early as possible in order to ensure that the results are back in time for when you need them.

- Ensuring that you have the capacity to handle emergencies, first by building up some slack into your schedule if you can do that. Should something happen, you will then have time to catch up on the delay that occurs. Second, by identifying who is available for help if needed.

- Making sure you plan your work in advance as much as you can, for example by reserving slots for specific matters (paperwork, teaching sessions, important meetings) as these may impose constraints onto your schedule. Arranging for cross-cover when needed.

Tools that you may use to support this

As well as discussing how you organise yourself, you could enrich your answer by mentioning the tools that you use to manage your work. These may include:

- PDA to keep track of patients
- Spreadsheet or word processor, e.g. for lists
- Electronic diary
- Secretary – this allows you to sell your team-playing abilities.

Formulating an answer

A good answer will consist of a three or four points discussed in separate paragraphs/sections, each of which should contain a personal example in order to avoid simply listing the same items as everyone else. For example, instead of saying "I make a list of patients and prioritise them. I delegate tasks to nurses and juniors, etc.", you can present a more developed and personal answer by saying something along the following lines:

> "...Before the ward round I prepare a list of all patients containing their basic details, diagnosis and summary management plan. After the ward round I have a short discussion with the other team members to agree how we can share the work. Following this I prioritise my own tasks in relation to their degree of urgency. I make sure that I request all blood tests and book diagnostic tests straight after the ward round so that the results can come back as early as possible. I update my job list throughout the day to take account of developments.
>
> During my attachment in Elderly Care, I had to prepare a lot of paperwork for discharge plans and found it useful to allocate a specific slot every day to carry out all administrative tasks, usually before the ward round as I was least likely to be disturbed ..."

You can discuss the tools that you use either as a separate section in your answer or by mixing the information with your examples. Whenever you mention a tool, try to explain not just that it is useful but also why it is useful. For example, "I regularly use a PDA" is informative but if many people say that then there is little information to distinguish between all of you. You could rephrase this statement as follows:

> "...I regularly use a PDA. As well as helping me keep the information in one place, it enables me to have rapid access to all essential information without having to carry pieces of paper in my pocket. It also helps me to be more efficient by giving me access to other forms of electronic information such as drug dosages ..."

8.21 How do you handle stress?

This is another generic question where there is a risk of giving the same answer as hundreds of other candidates and, therefore, where you need to illustrate each point with personal examples in order to stand out. The marking schedule for this question will typically be rewarding:

- The variety of ways in which you can deal with stress
- Your ability to identify that you are getting stressed
- Your ability to show the relevance of the information to your work (i.e. by bringing personal examples, and, in the case of your hobbies, by explaining what you gain from them).

Many candidates fall into the trap of concentrating on their hobbies. In reality, interviewers will be looking for a broad range of ways of dealing with stress, including in the workplace. Note that the question does not explicitly ask how you recognise that you are stressed; however, it is a sad fact that many marking schemes allocate marks for relevant information that is not always explicitly requested. When in doubt, you should aim to provide an answer which is as complete as possible by looking beyond the exact wording of the question and providing other relevant information. If your interviewers are helpful, they may prompt you for that information; others have higher expectations and may not be so kind.

Handling stress

There are different types of stress to which you may be exposed both at work and in your personal life. Depending on the type of stress that you are facing, you will react and cope differently. This may include:

For stress caused by busy situations (e.g. being overworked):
- Taking a step back
- Remaining calm
- Organising your work, prioritising and delegating
- Trying to anticipate difficult periods and planning accordingly
- Taking appropriate breaks
- Breaking tasks off into smaller, more manageable chunks
- Asking for help from your colleagues
- Communicating well with others (e.g. maintaining momentum in a team to ensure full coordination)
- Managing others' expectations (for example, if you are prioritising, inevitably someone's main priority will become bottom of your list. Not managing their expectations would potentially result in a conflict).

For stress of a more emotional nature (e.g. difficulty in dealing with negative issues such as personality clashes, patient deaths, high expectations from others, feeling of powerlessness)
- Sharing your problems with colleagues
- Discussing problems with your friends and family.

For general stress (e.g. accumulation of fatigue)
- Socialising with colleagues or friends
- Having time for yourself, hobbies, centres of interest outside medicine.

Rather than simply list some of the above items, you should focus your answer on your personal experience, explaining how you deal with a range of different situations that you commonly face in the workplace. Since the question is not specifically relating to the workplace, you may also mix some information relating to other settings if you feel that they are appropriate.

Example of an effective answer

"I deal with stress differently depending on the situation. For example, during my on-calls, I often have to deal with multiple admissions on my own, some of which can take a long time to handle. In such circumstances, I find it very useful to take stock of the situation once the most urgent matters have been attended to. This ensures that I remain in control of the situation and do not miss any important tasks. If I feel that an issue may cause problems later on, I keep in touch with my Registrar so that he is aware of the situation and able to provide input as needed. I also work closely with the nurses because they are invaluable in getting some of the tasks done very efficiently and often provide very useful information that I can use to make more informed decisions for our patients. When I am very busy, I try to take a short break to have a coffee. I find that having regular breaks really helps to keep me focused.

When I worked in Elderly Care, I found many relatives had unreasonably high expectations; this could be stressful at times. Although I could see that they had their family member's best interest at heart, I found they were often keen to blame the medical profession for a patient's lifestyle excesses, poor adherence to treatment or general poor health. This created a sometimes very negative and stressful atmosphere. Generally speaking, I was able to deal with this because I felt that they reacted in this way as a result of a natural concern for their relative. If ever I feel that the tension is rising or that I may be using a more aggressive tone of voice, I take some time out to rethink my approach or to consult a colleague on the best approach. It can be very useful to discuss problems with colleagues as it provides an opportunity to share the problem with someone else but also to understand how *they* deal with similar issues. Often, we both learn from these conversations and I have found that, since I have been talking to them in this way, they have started to do the same with me. This has led to better team working, which has further reduced stress.

I think that the key to a stress-free life is to make sure that you are properly conditioned to deal with problems. I have often found that I react much more calmly to problems when I have had the opportunity to relax outside work. Personally, I enjoy playing sport with friends, particularly cricket. I also enjoy reading books such as crime novels and history books. I find that, by combining group and personal activities, I strike a good balance in my leisure time which then makes it easier to deal with stress generally.

Friends and colleagues often comment that I am a relaxed individual but I know that stress is beginning to affect me if I start to find it difficult to think straight or become irritable or disorganised. When I recognise this I make sure that I set aside some valuable relaxation time, usually in the evening, to stop letting the stress get to me."

8.22 How do you recognise that you are stressed?

Ways in which you can recognise that you are stressed include:

Behavioural effects

- Feeling tired, tense, irritable or anxious
- Tendency to drink more or smoke more (not to excess though!)
- Poor concentration. Becoming forgetful. Making small/silly mistakes
- Difficulty in dealing calmly with everyday pressures
- Loss of appetite/too much appetite
- Working shorter or longer hours
- Poor time management or punctuality
- Shorter fuse. Increased tension and conflict with colleagues or patients.

Physical effects

- Lower resistance to infection
- Raised heart rate
- Aching neck and shoulder
- Headaches
- Insomnia

Note: this is not a clinical question on the manifestations of stress, so there is no need to become highly detailed by mentioning some recognised but less appealing symptoms such as "blurred vision" or "dizziness", which could impair your ability to be safe at work.

Avoid listing a number of points as this will make your answer bland. Draw upon real situations where you became stressed in the past, explain how you identify that you were stressed and then briefly explain how you dealt with that stress. The emphasis should be on stress recognition rather than stress resolution here, though you should ensure that you mention both, as both are likely to appear in the marking scheme.

8.23 Give an example of a stressful situation in which you have been involved

This question is testing your ability to deal with pressure and stress by means of an example. Through discussing the example, you will be expected to explain which demands were made on you personally and how you coped/dealt with them.

Which examples can you discuss?

Try to choose a complex enough scenario where you were really stressed, otherwise you will struggle to explain the issue convincingly and to demonstrate your full skills set. This may include situations where you had to:

- Deal with several tasks at the same time, e.g. several emergencies, urgent requests or tasks with tight deadlines
- Do something that was unfamiliar and which you were under pressure to deliver quickly
- Deal with a difficult or abusive patient who was taking your time, putting you behind in the rest of your work
- Work with a colleague who was difficult or unhelpful
- Deal with the workload of one or several absent colleagues with little or no senior availability
- Negotiate with a colleague who disagreed with your approach, when you had little time to argue.

Delivering the answer

Once you have settled on one example, identify the skills and behaviours that you exhibited to deal with the situation and avoid/deal with your stress. For example, if you had to deal with a multitasking situation then you will inevitably have to mention:

- How you prioritised the patients and shared the workload with colleagues to resolve the situation
- How you ensured that you maintained good communication
- How you gained support from seniors
- How, maybe, you negotiated with colleagues to make room for small breaks for yourself and others.

If you had to deal with a difficult patient, you will talk about how you ensured you remained calm, used all your communication skills to establish a rapport and deal with the patient, and maybe involved other team members to help you out.

Don't lose sight of the fact that the question is about the stress incurred during the scenario and not just about the situation itself. This means that you must go into detail about what demands, pressure and stress you faced, what *you* did, and how it helped resolve the problem and reduce your stress level.

Concluding the answer

Conclude your answer by explaining what happened at the end and, if appropriate, how you relaxed when you went back home (had a bath, relaxed with family, played table tennis with friends, etc.) to provide a complete answer.

If the situation provided an opportunity to learn from it and develop new skills and behaviours, then you should mention it. For example, after dealing with a difficult patient, you might have debriefed with a senior colleague and discussed alternative approaches. You might even have agreed to develop your skills further by going on a communication skills course. Similarly, after dealing with multiple emergencies or a difficult on-call, you might have sought advice from senior colleagues and learnt about other ways of working. Basically, if there is an opportunity to learn, make sure you mention and present yourself as someone who is always trying to improve and develop.

If the stress was due to a systemic problem (e.g. an inefficient system, the absence of the right equipment, the short-notice unavailability of staff) then you could also explain how you tried to change the system once the event was over (e.g. introducing a new pro forma, arranging a team meeting to discuss the problem) as a means to prevent the stressful situation from recurring.

8.24	Describe a situation when you have used a holistic approach in managing a patient

What the interviewers are looking for

The question asks you to discuss how you have used a holistic approach as part of a real-life scenario. In your answer, you will be expected to describe, through the use of a specific personal example, how you identified and addressed the physical, social and psychological needs of a patient.

This may seem like stating the obvious but it frames the question and without considering the answer in this way you will not score well. The key to this question is really to find a good example that enables you to demonstrate your experience and ability in applying all three aspects in the management of a single patient.

Note that the question asks for a clinical situation. It does not mean you have to go into vast clinical detail but simply that it must be related to a patient at work, rather than, say, a friend whom you might have dealt with.

Examples you can discuss

Your example must describe your care of a patient and must include all of the aforementioned areas. This could include:

- An elderly patient who needed to be discharged
- A patient to whom you broke bad news
- A patient whose lifestyle was being affected by their condition
- A patient who was finding it difficult to cope with their diagnosis
- A homeless patient
- A patient with multiple conditions ranging from psychological to physical.

Use the STAR structure (see 5.2)

Situation/Task	Describe the type of patient and how they presented to you.
Action	Explain how you recognised and addressed the patient's different needs.
Result/Reflect	Explain how the patient was helped with your approach (grateful, much improved lifestyle, got a new job and sorted themselves out, etc.). Explain what you feel you did well and, if prompted, what you could have done better.

Try to be as practical as you can, describing what you actually did to address the patient's needs. Too many candidates offer statements such as: "I identified the patient's psychological needs and addressed them appropriately".

This only explains what needs you identified, but it would be interesting to know what those needs exactly were and how they were addressed. For example, the patient may have had a need for psychological support; consequently, you discussed support groups and gave the patient leaflets to read and websites to visit.

The different needs

Physical needs
Describe the physical needs of the patient and how you addressed them. In this section try to give just enough detail to clearly communicate that you were competent but do not overdo it on the clinical detail – this is not the purpose of the question. In some cases, your answers could even be as simple as referring the patient to a specialist or to a senior colleague. All that matters is that you have addressed the needs in a sensible manner.

Social needs
Describe the social needs of the patient. Did they live on their own? Did they have family? Could their family cope with the burden? Did they need community support? What about financial aspects? Did they need advice about claiming benefits? Were there charities that could help? Did their home require special adjustments? Did you enlist the help of some members of the multidisciplinary team to sort out some of the issues (care workers, occupational therapist, community nurses, etc.)? Did you provide leaflets?

Psychological needs
Describe the psychological needs of the patient. Did they need support in coming to terms with a difficult diagnosis or chronic illness? Did they need counselling? Did they require a referral to a psychiatrist? Did you arrange for the patient to get in touch with charities? Did you spend some time counselling them yourself? Did you address this issue with the relatives? Did the relatives need counselling too?

8.25 Describe a time when you had to deal with a sceptical patient

This is another question asking for an example and which you will therefore need to answer using the STAR approach (see 5.2). This question is primarily about communication, the respect of others and, in some cases, teamwork (e.g. if you need to involve input from other people to help you resolve the situation).

What the interviewers are looking for

The main criteria that the interviewers will be looking for include:

Communication
- Listening to the patient's point of view, exploring the patient's concerns and addressing any underlying issues. For example, if they distrust conventional medicine, you should investigate why.

- Communication with the patient in a way they can understand (basic English if needed, interpreter, diagrams) and that they have time to digest the information and ask questions to you or others.

- Ensuring that the patient receives all the information that you can give them. This could be through the involvement of other professionals (for example, by involving another colleague, a nurse or referring to a suitable specialist) or by giving a leaflet.

Teamwork
Asking a senior colleague or other member of the team for advice on how you should handle the situation or asking them to intervene if necessary

Respect for patient's autonomy
The patient has the right to make a decision for themselves. If, in your example, your patient still disagreed with you despite your best efforts, don't panic – this may be a powerful example; what matters is how you dealt with it. It is a patient's right to disagree and your duty to accept that they can do so. In such cases, it is important to have demonstrated that they understood what the consequences might be for them and what other options were available. It is also important to mention that you documented the essence of the conversation and the decision.

Examples you can discuss

There are many reasons for a patient to be sceptical. Here are a few examples that you may have encountered recently:

- They do not trust you for one reason or another. Maybe they have prior bad experiences with friends or relatives that would make them doubt your word.

- They may have gained information from the media (for example, through TV, newspapers or the Internet) that gives them a different perspective.

- They may be medically aware, i.e. they are scientists or linked to the medical profession. They require more information than your average patient.

- They may have personal beliefs (against conventional treatment for example) or simply a language problem.

- They have a problem with you (e.g. a male patient being suspicious of a female doctor, a patient trusting older doctors only, etc.).

- Your explanations or proposed management options may be different to their expectations.

Once you have found the right example, describing the situation is fairly straightforward using the STAR technique (see 5.2).

8.26 Outline a time when you had to support a colleague with a work-related problem

Although the topic raised by the question is that of a colleague in difficulty, this is not a question about how to deal with a difficult colleague or an unsafe colleague. It is really a question about support, and therefore communication and teamwork, so you should ensure that your answer focuses on these two skills.

The type of situations where you may have needed to support a colleague with a work-related problem may include:

A busy colleague who finds it hard to find time to study

You would discuss the situation with the colleague and perhaps offer to take on some of their tasks when appropriate to relieve them from the pressure they face. If they are busy because they are not very efficient, you may offer to help them out by showing them how they can plan and organise their work better (making sure you are not patronising them in doing so). If you are also studying for exams, you may consider supporting them by pairing up with them to revise together. If you have already passed the exam they are studying for, you could organise informal teaching/support sessions to help them out.

A colleague who lacks knowledge or experience and struggles

First of all you must make sure your colleague is not performing tasks beyond their level of competence. You can encapsulate this in your answer by stating that your priority would be to ensure the highest standard of patient care and safety. Many people have small knowledge-based sticking points that they feel stupid asking about because they feel they should know them. If this is the case, you could give a brief explanation or tutorial and then explain how you learned this and if there are good books or web resources that you use when you are stuck. This encourages them to try to look things up themselves the next time they are stuck.

If the issue is the need to learn a practical skill, see if it is something you can go over in a skills lab together – you may find that there is a simple step that is being forgotten, and this is a very easy environment to iron this out. If it is more complex, you could recommend the course that you did to learn the skill or set up some ward-based mentorship for the skill. If you know that the task in question is being performed then you could encourage your colleague to be there when it happens and ideally adjust the rota so that they have an opportunity to reinforce their learning of that skill with practical experience.

The basis of your answer is that you would support your colleague, making sure that they are not exposed to situations where they feel stupid or dangerous, and encourage them to improve their knowledge or skills to overcome any deficiency.

A colleague in a personality clash with another colleague

Dealing with personality clashes from an external perspective is always dangerous because you risk making matters worse by appearing to take sides. Supporting your colleague may consist of listening to them and allowing them to vent their frustration so they know that they can share their problem with someone else. This may help your colleague put things in perspective and discuss the issue with their colleague directly. If the clash is with someone more senior then you may encourage your colleague to discuss the problem with another senior colleague whom they trust (e.g. a consultant, their educational supervisor). Essentially, you would ensure that you are there for them without necessarily getting directly involved yourself in resolving the matter. You are *supporting* your colleague, not *replacing* them.

A colleague who finds it hard to remain motivated in their job

You must never lose sight of the fact that you are supporting your colleague and not seeking to dictate a course of action to them. Supporting them may involve sitting down with them to help them understand why they are not motivated. Perhaps they are not getting enough support from senior colleagues in which case you may want to encourage them to raise the issue with their educational supervisor. Perhaps they are doing an attachment in a specialty that does not interest them, in which case you may wish to discuss with them how they can make the attachment more interesting or help them understand the importance or advantages of their current job in their long-term career plan; perhaps you would encourage them to get involved in a project such as an audit to give them a sense of purpose.

A colleague who is being bullied by a senior colleague

Bullying is not acceptable in any environment but, whilst you may want to try to resolve the issue yourself, you should try to take the part of a supportive friend and aim to maintain an objective view. Direct involvement on your part should be a last resort.

Your support should begin by simply listening to your colleague and helping them think about the problem rather than getting involved yourself – it will help you to establish their side of the story. If you felt that patient care was being compromised and that your colleague was unable to deal with the problem then you would need to raise the matter with a senior colleague. If you can, avoid discussing topics involving drink, drugs or bullying unless the interviewers specifically ask you about them (we will see how to handle difficult colleagues later on) as this takes the attention away from the support towards your colleague and it may lead to answers which are potentially controversial.

Note that the question is asking for a work-related problem and not a personal problem. However, in some circumstances, the two will be inextricably linked (i.e. problems such as a sick child, marital problems or even train delays may have an impact on work-related performance). You can therefore mention in your answer how you sought to support your colleague in relation to more personal problems, but only to the extent that they are impacting on their work and providing they do not form the main thread of your answer; otherwise your answer will be off-topic and your score will be accordingly low.

Delivering the answer

Since the question is asking for a specific example, you should make sure that you do not speak generically about how you would support a colleague but that you provide an example of a specific situation.

You should structure your answer using the STAR approach (see 5.2), explaining first the nature of the problem from your colleague's point of view (i.e. setting out why he/she was in need of support), explaining how you supported him, and how the story ended (hopefully your actions led to a positive outcome).

Be prepared to answer a follow-up question on what you could have done better. There is no need to volunteer this information unless they request it explicitly when probing.

8.27 What skills or personal attributes do you possess that will make you a good trainee in this specialty?

This is a very broad question which leaves many candidates perplexed simply because they don't know where to start.

Where are the marks?

For this type of question, the marking scheme will reward:

- Your understanding of the specialty and the training
- Your ability to list skills and attributes relevant to the specialty
- Your ability to demonstrate, with full use of your personal experience, that you possess those skills and attributes
- The clarity of your answer (which will come from the structure of your answer and the concise nature of your examples).

Which skills and attributes can you mention?

The answer very much depends on the Person Specification for your specialty and grade. When you face such a question, you can talk about pretty much what you want, providing you respect the following rules:

- Ensure that the skills and attributes mentioned cover a wide enough spectrum. You should consult the Person Specification to understand the requirements that your interviewers will be testing.

- Choose a maximum of four skills and attributes. Although the Person Specification may cover a lot more than four, you cannot possibly talk about all of them in 2 minutes; otherwise you will remain very superficial. Give priority to those for which you can more easily demonstrate your suitability, experience and strengths.

- Choose skills and attributes which are strongly linked to the specialty and order them in decreasing order of importance. For example, being empathetic and a good listener are both important in most specialties but, in some specialties, other skills are more prominently used. In Paediatrics, Psychiatry and Oncology, empathy will therefore rank higher than in specialties such as surgery, where empathy may be preceded in the list by the ability to work well under pressure or learn new techniques. In medicine, empathy may be preceded by your problem-solving ability. A good starting point to measure the relative importance of the different skills is to look at the order in which they are listed in the Person Specification.

- Structure your answer on a skill by skill basis. Mention one skill/attribute and explain why it is important for the specialty. Give examples from your experience to back up your claims.

- Make sure that you are specific in the description of the skills and attributes that you choose to present. For example, "I am a good communicator" is vague. A punchier statement would be "I am a good communicator and, in particular, I am very effective at dealing with conflict between other team members or situations where I need to negotiate with others." The more specific you are, the more impact you will have and the easier it will be to find suitable examples to illustrate your purpose.

- If you can, try to group several skills in one point if they are related. For example, you may want to say that you are good at making decisions, that you call for help when necessary and that you are a good team player. These could constitute three different points but you could also raise all of them in one single point, with a sentence such as: "I am very good at making decisions when faced with difficult situations and I am always prepared to ask for help, if required. I am also very good at implementing my decisions by communicating with the relevant colleagues and delegating responsibilities appropriately" (you can then follow this with an example). This approach gives more body to your answer.

Examples of structures for different specialties

Most surgical specialties (and specialties with procedures)

Example 1
- Good manual dexterity and hand-eye coordination
- Good ability to keep calm under pressure and make sensible decisions (including seeking help from others if necessary)
- Very good at engaging with patients, explaining procedures and providing reassurance when necessary
- Good team-working abilities, in particular: good relationships with all team members, good ability to communicate with others to coordinate activities such as theatre lists and teaching sessions, and good ability to deal with potential conflicts sensitively.

Example 2
- Patient, able to remain calm under pressure and to take initiative in challenging situations
- Able to make decisions and resolve complex issues, calling for help if required
- Good at engaging with people at all levels, whether they are patients, junior colleagues or senior colleagues
- Committed to hard work, enjoy volunteering for new projects and willing to learn from own experience.

145

Most medical specialties

Example 1
- Good communication skills, able to address a wide range of people with different levels of understanding and different cultural backgrounds
- Confident in addressing complex issues and able to think laterally to find solutions to problems
- Very organised, able to work well with others and to use the team appropriately in order to get the work done
- Able to deal with stress in difficult situations and to call for advice or help when required.

Example 2
- Relate easily to a wide range of people, whether they are patients or doctors, both in the clinical and non-clinical environment
- Caring and supportive. Able to show empathy towards patients but also towards colleagues, volunteering to help when required
- Good analytical skills and good ability to make decisions both independently and with senior advice, if required
- Organised and able to deal with difficult situations through teamwork, self-discipline and tenacity.

Anaesthesia
- Vigilant even in situations of low activity. Able to respond quickly and efficiently when a problem occurs
- Very organised and thorough. Able to work well under pressure, remain calm and take appropriate decisions, calling for help if necessary
- Good team player and, in particular, able to communicate well with colleagues at all levels. Not afraid to discuss problems if necessary, even with seniors
- Empathic, good listener and able to engage quickly with patients.

Psychiatry
- Good ability to communicate and work well within a team, both with immediate colleagues, and with members of various multidisciplinary teams
- Able to cooperate with others to achieve results. Non-judgemental and aware of impact of own actions on others
- Empathic and supportive, particularly towards vulnerable people. Good at reassuring people, dealing with difficult issues sensitively and managing expectations.
- Able to make safe decisions under pressure and to deal with stress. Good at planning and therefore very aware of possible dangers and conflicts that may arise.

Obstetrics & Gynaecology / Paediatrics
- Good listener, able to engage with patients, to reassure and empathise
- Good at dealing sensitively with difficult issues and breaking bad news

- Quick thinking and able to deal well with pressure. Good at making safe decisions quickly, asking for help from senior colleagues if required.
- Good at collaborating with a wide range of people. Sensitive to the needs of the various members of the team.

Delivering your answer

You can see from the above that many of the same skills and attributes are common in different answers. After all, there is only limited choice. You will not be judged on how different your answer sounds (i.e. you don't have to find some obscure skill to stand out) but on the completeness of your answer and the way in which you illustrate the points that you are making.

Once you have made a point (which may consist of several statements as shown in each bullet point above), provide examples from your practice. It is best to avoid going into too much detail for the examples as you only have 20 to 30 seconds per point. This can be achieved either by sticking to one example per point, which you briefly describe without going into too much detail (otherwise you won't have much time for other points; or by listing several general situations where you may have demonstrated the skill in question, explaining briefly afterwards how you handled the situation

---

Example of an effective answer (partial – using one example only)

"I am patient, able to remain calm under pressure and to take the initiative in challenging situations. For example, recently I was confronted with an angry patient during one my shifts. I could see that he was becoming more agitated and as he had verbally threatened staff I was concerned about the risk of him becoming violent. I made sure that a nurse went to get some help whilst I talked to the patient to try and persuade him to calm down. It took a while, but by involving other members of the team appropriately and communicating I was able to obtain a positive outcome."

You can see that the example is only briefly expanded upon, almost as a teaser for the interviewers. Their next question is then likely to ask you to expand on the situation. Also, as this is only one point out of four, there is no time to dwell on the detail too much. The communication and teamwork aspects are emphasised just enough to make the point.

Example of an effective answer (partial – listing several examples)

"I feel that I am good at dealing sensitively with difficult issues. Over the past couple of years, I have had to break bad news to mothers who had ectopic pregnancies, to deal with sensitive private matters with patients who felt uncomfortable opening themselves up to a stranger and I was even confronted with a case of

---

child abuse. In all these situations, I was able to remain non-judgemental and to take my patients through their situation step by step, ensuring that I communicated empathically but efficiently, providing reassurance as appropriate and, if necessary, ensuring that they were supported by other appropriate members of the team.

Again, there is no time to go into any detail. What you are trying to achieve is a demonstration, to your panel, of where and how you use the skill stated, with a view that, if they are interested, they may ask for more detail about any particular example.

8.28 What are your main strengths?

This question is in fact the same one as 8.27. Your main strengths should be the skills and attributes that make you suitable for the specialty and there is therefore no reason why you should be providing a different answer. Other questions that can be answered in a similar fashion include:

- How would your colleagues describe you?
- What would your friends say about you?
- What would you like your consultant to write in your reference?
- If I looked at your multi-source feedback, what would it say? (Stay away from any negative feedback unless they ask)
- What makes you a good doctor?
- What would you like written in your obituary?

What if they only ask for a single strength?

It may be that the question is worded in the singular, i.e. "What would you consider to be your single biggest strength?" If this happens then the approach to the question is the same except that you will need to place your entire focus on just one of the four points that you would normally mention.

There is one trick though that will enable you to sell a bit more than just one point: it is to simply list a range of points in the first sentence before zooming in on the main point that you want to talk about. It would give something like:

"Well, I have many strengths including being organised, able to work well under pressure, being a good team player and a good colleague. However, if I had to choose a single strength, I would say that it is my ability to communicate well with people at all levels, even in conflicting situations." <then illustrate with examples>

8.29 | What is your main weakness?

This question is often a worry for candidates, who fear that they may sound too clichéd or uninteresting by using a weakness that the interviewers are likely to have heard several times that day.

What is this question about?

Contrary to some of the interview myths which circulate, this question is NOT about demonstrating that you are perfect and that you have no weaknesses. On the contrary, the interviewers will be testing your honesty, your insight, your ability to learn from your mistakes/problems and to develop as an individual. Rather like the question on a mistake that you made (see 8.17), they expect you to talk openly about your own failures: an honest doctor is a safe doctor whom patients and colleagues can trust. So, don't be afraid to be personal as this is the only way in which you can maximise your mark.

Where do people go wrong when answering this question?

The problem does not lie so much in the weakness that candidates choose to mention in their answer but in the way it is delivered. Most answers sound clichéd because candidates present the weakness in a simplistic, almost black and white, manner. A common answer is of the format: "I can't say 'no', but I am aware of it and I am working on it." In such an answer, there is no attempt to explain exactly how they are dealing with it. This makes the answer very standard and totally uninteresting.

There is also no real attempt to explain in any detail what the impact of the weakness on the candidate is, for instance by providing an example which would lift any ambiguity. The lack of example means that the interviewers are left to extrapolate from the basic statement made by the candidate in any way they like and the candidate therefore loses control over the way in which their message is received.

For example:
- "I can't say 'no'" may give the impression that you are weak
- "I have high expectations of others" may give the impression that you are a control freak and unfriendly.

How to choose a good weakness

There are three parameters that you need to consider to choose a suitable weakness:

- Make sure that it is one of your real weaknesses as you will be much more at ease talking about it in detail than if you make it up (answers which are faked tend to sound rehearsed, vague and clichéd).

- Choose a weakness that, in different circumstances, can be considered a strength. The strategy is to present the weakness as a strength which can sometimes become a problem.

- Choose a weakness that can be remedied. There are weaknesses which can be difficult to correct, such as being disorganised, or getting frustrated at certain events. These are best avoided.

Examples of weaknesses

There are numerous examples of weakness that you can use, some being more original and creative than others. It is important that you choose one that you are comfortable talking about, as most of the impact that you will have in delivering the answer rests in your tone of voice and general confidence.

If you are unsure as to which weakness to choose, try different examples and see which one sounds best. I have set out below a range of weaknesses that you may want to consider, listing their negative and positive interpretations, together with some means of dealing with them. See if they are true to your situation and, if they are, adapt them to match your situation, bringing your own examples into the answer.

Being a perfectionist
This answer is probably one of most quoted at interviews, and one which is least likely to make you sound credible. By itself, it is not a bad weakness to mention but the interviewers will have heard it so many times in one day that you may just be subconsciously penalised for your lack of originality. If you want to use the "perfectionist" answer, I would advise you to find a more specific slant to the weakness so that you do not present it under such a broad heading. Some of the weaknesses have a "perfectionist" slant to them but sound less clichéd.

Finding it difficult to say "no"
This is also a commonly given answer, but perhaps a little less clichéd than the "perfectionist" answer, primarily because it has more words to it and therefore the impact is softened. If you want to use this weakness, you will need to convey the meaning of not being able to say "no", without actually using that phrase. For example: "there are times where I take on so many simultaneous projects that it can be difficult to juggle them all." The meaning is the same, but the wording is a bit more original.

Positive: You are a good team player, a good colleague, and always willing to help.

Negative: You may take on too much work and get stressed, or fail to deliver on some projects (hopefully minor ones!).

What you can do about it:
- Learn to become more assertive (more experience, course)
- Learn to manage colleagues' expectations (so that they are okay about you saying "no")
- Work with colleagues to help them find alternative solutions
- Be more realistic about your ability to deliver and more open with colleagues about issues
- Be more proactive in delegating to others so that you can say "yes" without having to take on everything yourself.

Having high standards and a tendency to expect others to follow the same standards as you
Positive: Being driven, you have achieved a lot and you deliver results to your team above their expectations. You have also encouraged others in your team to achieve and they did well as a result. You are seen as a good motivator and a "doer".

Negative: Some of your colleagues may not be able to follow your pace. You are trying to impose methods and principles which they may not adhere to and this may cause friction at times (i.e. you risk being seen as controlling).

What you can do about it:
- Learn to be a bit more flexible with colleagues. Take the time to know them. It may give you ideas about how you can approach them.
- Ensure that all team members have been trained in the skills you are expecting them to perform.
- Be more open-minded in your approach and accept that others may have ideas which are as good as, if not better than, yours.

Having a direct style of communication
This weakness is not suitable for specialties where communication is an ultra-essential skill (such as Paediatrics, Psychiatry and any fundamentally holistic specialty). However, if addressed properly, it can be used successfully for a wide range of specialties, from surgical specialties to general medical specialties and even specialties such as Public Health.

Positive: People know where they stand with you; they know that if they ask for your opinion they will get an answer which they can use towards their own thinking process. Generally, you find it easy to be trusted because people know that, if there is an issue, you will discuss it openly.

Negative: There are times when more subtlety and diplomacy is required, and you may encounter situations where communicating too openly may cause friction.

What you can do about it:
- Learn to appreciate the impact of your communication on others
- Learn to recognise when you can be yourself and when you need to soften your style
- Seek guidance from seniors; perhaps go on a course.

Finding it difficult to delegate
This weakness is the result of lack of experience of working in a delegation environment. This lack of experience, coupled with the fear that you may lose control of the situation, leads to your taking over the situation.

Positive: You deliver consistently good results and, in an environment where most people rotate frequently, it can be an asset not to overload new team members until they have established their ability.

Negative: People may see you as someone distant (sometimes). Also, by trying to do everything yourself, you end up having too much on your plate, with a risk of getting stressed.

What you can do about it:
- Be more attentive to juniors and find opportunities to delegate
- Get to know your colleagues early on so that you find it easier to trust them and therefore delegate
- Discuss with your seniors and/or go on a course.

Tendency to take criticism or negative outcomes personally
This weakness can work well if you have the right type of personality. I would not recommend it for surgical specialties though where interviewers can be less forgiving about a lack of confidence than in other specialties.

Positive: Taking things personally pushes you to act on problems quickly.

Negative: Being over-negative may make you appear under-confident (and miserable)

What you can do about it:
- Discuss with colleagues and see how they deal with criticism, complaints and negative outcomes
- Use every incident as an opportunity to learn.

Getting too involved with patients
This would refer to situations where patients have many issues and where you find it difficult to put a stop to a consultation for fear of missing something out or upsetting the patient.

Positive: You are thorough and caring.

<u>Negative</u>: You can overrun and/or get stressed

<u>What you can do about it</u>:
- Learn to become gently assertive
- Discuss with colleagues to understand how they do it.

Getting too attached to patients
This refers to situations where you are struggling to maintain the professional barrier in your dealings with a patient and push the empathy to a point where it personally affects you psychologically.

<u>Positive</u>: You are caring and empathetic.

<u>Negative</u>: You get stressed.

<u>What you can do about it</u>:
- Learn through experience to keep the appropriate distance
- Discuss with colleagues/seniors.

Taking your worries home with you
This refers to situations where you finish your work and feel the need to double-check things when you get home or keep worrying about whether your instructions will be followed once you have left. In some cases, this may result in your having to call the ward once home, or even to stay late to ensure that things are done properly.

<u>Positive</u>: You are thorough and conscientious.

<u>Negative</u>: You may get stressed or even irritate others, who feel you don't trust them. It may also interfere with your social/private life.

<u>What you can do about it</u>:
- Optimise your communication with colleagues so that you can be sure they know what needs to be done
- Discuss with colleagues how they deal with it
- In the more extreme cases, call the ward once only when back home so that you then have your entire evening clear afterwards.

All these are examples, which will work well if they are explained in a personal manner. There are other approaches that you can adopt, but which, in my experience, are less successful. These include:

- Using a weakness which is not linked to personality but to something practical, such as lack of research. Most marking schemes would be based around a personality-based weakness and therefore using a more practical weakness may score lower. If you have any doubt, or if you are really keen to talk about a non-personality-related weakness, then there is no harm in asking the interviewers whether they want a personality-based weakness or whether you can use something relating to your training.

- Using a weakness which is in the past and already resolved. This does not answer the question, which is "What is your main weakness?". Using an old weakness would not demonstrate that you have any insight into your current behaviours and therefore may score lower. Under the new ST interview system experience shows that playing safe rarely pays off. There is a benefit in taking risks.

Structure to answer the question

There are many ways in which you can answer this question; however, having heard thousands of people answering this question both in my experience of interviewing and in my coaching experience, I have found the following structure to be one of the most effective:

Step 1:	**Quick positive introduction** to place a positive context on the weakness (this must be no more than 15 seconds or so, otherwise you will give the impression that you are avoiding the question).
Step 2:	**State the weakness and explain the negative impact it has**. In doing so, ensure that you use words which do not make the weakness sound awful. "I can't delegate effectively" sounds bad, but "I sometimes find it difficult to delegate, particularly when working with new junior colleagues" is more specific and more realistic too.
Step 3:	**Give a specific example** of a situation which illustrates the weakness. Spend some time on this section. The purpose of the example is to remove any doubt in the interviewers' mind about the seriousness of the weakness.
Step 4:	**Explain what you learnt from that situation.** This will enable the interviewers to visualise exactly how reflective you can be. This, together with the next step, is one of the most important parts of the answer.
Step 5:	**Explain how you attempt to deal with the weakness generally.** This will ensure that the interviewers tick the marking box which says "Takes concrete steps to remedy the weakness".

Example of an effective answer

It would take hundreds of pages to illustrate how each weakness can be discussed; however, once you have read the following sample answer, you will get the idea of how the above structure can be applied and you will have no problem adapting it to your own experience and circumstances. I have chosen the weakness of "taking on too much" to demonstrate how you can build the answer using the different steps stated above.

Step 1	"I have always been an ambitious person and, as a result, I always show a lot of enthusiasm in getting involved in all sorts of projects. If you look at my CV, you will see that I have achieved a lot, not only in terms of clinical experience, but also in terms of audit and teaching experience.
Step 2	However, there are times where I have been a little too greedy and became involved in too many projects at once, as a result of which I either placed myself under too much pressure, or I had to arrange an extension of the deadline.
Step 3	One example that springs to mind is a situation which arose last year, when, as well as doing 1:4 on-calls and studying hard for my Part 1 membership exams, I had agreed to deliver quarterly lectures to medical students, volunteered to do some number-crunching for my consultant's research project and also agreed to do two audits, one of which I was keen to lead throughout. After two months, I could see that I would never be able to complete all this before I moved to my next post and so I had to go back to my consultant to explain that I could only do one of the audits.
Step 4	I felt I had let down my colleagues in this particular instance, but it made me realise how crucial it is to be aware of your own capacities and that, although you may look good when you accept a project, it can cause problems if you don't deliver. On reflection, I also feel that I could have delivered as expected if I had thought about involving someone else when there was still time to do so, such as a medical student, who could have made a start on collecting the data.
Step 5	I have become very aware of the problems associated with getting involved in too many projects and the impact both on myself and on other people. As a result, I try my best to think carefully before launching into new projects (without curbing my own enthusiasm, of course). I also try to involve others more when appropriate, which has the advantage of getting juniors involved in new projects too."

9 Academic & Clinical Governance questions

Questions on academic activities (e.g. teaching, research) or on clinical governance are increasingly common at CT and ST interviews. These can be generic (e.g. "What is clinical governance?") or specific (e.g. "How does risk management affect your daily practice?").

They are generally easier to prepare for than the more personal questions addressed in previous chapters because they are factual and therefore rely, to a large extent, on information that you will have learnt before the interview. However, to achieve a high mark, repeating information learnt by heart will not be enough; you will be expected to reflect on your own experience and provide a more personal slant to the issues raised. This chapter will provide you with essential information that you may need at your interview.

In some academic and clinical governance stations, you may be asked to discuss a paper that you have read recently; I would therefore advise you to read the journals appropriate for your preferred specialty before the interview so that you can approach such a question confidently.

On occasion, the interviewers may ask you to critically appraise a specific paper, which you will be given a reasonable amount of time to read prior to the interview (anything between 20 and 60 minutes). To perform well, you will obviously have in mind a process to critically appraise a paper; this chapter will also help you considerably with this task.

9.1   Tell us about your teaching experience

This is a fairly straightforward question, where you can easily shine provided that you give an answer which goes beyond the obvious day-to-day informal teaching experience that you may have. Indeed, most marking schemes allocate very few marks for informal teaching experience and reward candidates who show more initiative and enthusiasm towards teaching. To optimise your marks, you will need to provide as much information as possible in each of the following sections.

Section 1: Actual teaching experience

You can structure this section in two ways:

Structure 1 Different types of teaching	Structure 2 Different types of groups taught
<ul><li>Informal teaching</li><li>Lectures (big groups)</li><li>Workshops (incl. ALS)</li><li>Presentations<ul><li>– Departmental</li><li>– Grand round</li><li>– Regional</li></ul></li></ul>	<ul><li>Undergraduates</li><li>FYs & STs</li><li>Others (e.g. nurses, GPs, paramedics)</li><li>Teaching outside medicine (if you do some)</li></ul>

Whatever structure you choose, you will need to describe the extent of your teaching experience, covering:

- the types of groups you have taught
- the teaching methods you used (e.g. simulation, role play)
- the types of topics that you taught (e.g. clinical knowledge/skills, procedures, history taking, breaking bad news, etc.).

Most marking schemes allocate further marks if the candidate has organised teaching sessions and/or written teaching material from scratch (as opposed to simply delivering teaching to a group of people). Therefore, if you have shown initiative in organising teaching groups or in writing your own lectures, make sure that you highlight it clearly.

Describe how you plan your teaching to meet the needs of the learners and how you use questions and answers to monitor their progress and understanding. Do you use any form of MCQ/quiz at the end to assess their learning? Do you evaluate the process of your teaching (i.e. how it went and what you could do to improve)?

Section 2: Teaching courses attended

If you have attended any teaching courses, mention them. They will form part of the marking scheme and will reflect the care that you demonstrate in developing your skills.

Do not limit yourself to stating that you went to a course; explain also what you gained from it and how it helped you improve your teaching skills. Remember: the more personal your answer is, the stronger its impact.

Section 3: Feedback

- **Collecting feedback**
  The interviewers will want to know that you take teaching seriously and that you make an effort to find out what others think of your performance. This will portray the image of someone who is keen to improve constantly. In this section, you should therefore explain how you seek feedback from those you teach. Hopefully, this will be through formal means such as a questionnaire being distributed at the end of the teaching session. However, if you have not collected formal feedback, then you can of course talk about how you collect informal feedback from colleagues.

  Generally speaking, introducing qualitative feedback into your answer (e.g. "The vast majority of the students enjoyed it because ...") will have a better effect than presenting quantitative feedback (e.g. "All of the medical students gave me 9/10").

- **Nature of the feedback**
  As well as explaining that you collect feedback, you can push the answer further by stating what that feedback is (limiting yourself to the positive feedback). Sell yourself by stating what others think of your teaching (e.g. that you are very organised, very good at expressing complex ideas in simple terms, good at anticipating the audience's needs).

Section 4: Why you enjoy teaching and future plans

The marking schedule will allow for your enthusiasm and commitment. You should therefore emphasise how important teaching is in medicine and explain what you enjoy about it (see question 9.2 for ideas). If you have specific plans for the future, e.g. taking up a medical education degree or getting involved with Royal College teaching and training initiatives, then you should mention them.

9.2 Why do you enjoy teaching?

There are many things that one can enjoy about teaching and you will most likely be able to come up with your own reasons. Generally speaking, you may wish to consider the following points:

- You get personal satisfaction from participating in the development of your colleagues and the feedback that you have been getting certainly shows that people appreciate your input.

- It helps the team bond together. By spending time with your colleagues away from the pressures of your daily routine, you can build better working relationships, which in turn translates into better patient care and a good atmosphere at work (well, sometimes anyway!).

- You can learn a lot from teaching others. Not only do they force you to know your topic in depth (they might ask all sorts of questions at the end of the session) but you also learn through the preparation that you do. For example, to prepare for a teaching session, you may need to go over your textbooks again, reading journals, looking up guidelines, etc.

Back up each of these points (and any others you may have decided upon) with personal examples. For example, for the third point (learning during the preparation of the teaching session), take the specific example of a recent talk that you prepared and explain what you learnt (or consolidated) as a result.

9.3   What are the qualities of a good teacher?

This is a general question (i.e. not explicitly asking about your own qualities) but, nevertheless, the marking schedule will expect you to go beyond the general approach, to discuss your own skills and experience. I suggest that you answer this question in two sections:

Section 1 – General answer

Describe what makes a good teacher, explaining why each quality is important. To make the answer more interesting, you can draw upon your experience, illustrating your answer by talking about how you were particularly well taught or inspired by a specific consultant or speaker. Here are some of the key qualities of a good teacher:

- Sets appropriate, specific and challenging goals
- Has a clear plan to achieve his/her goal and has a clear delivery of his/her topic
- Involves the students, continually assesses the learning and provides feedback
- Is positive and encouraging
- Is able to promote enthusiasm in his/her students
- Is able to adapt to the students and alter his/her methods accordingly
- Is resourceful and adopts a problem-solving approach
- Respects his/her students
- Gathers feedback and reflects on negative feedback.

Section 2 – Personal experience

Explain that these are qualities which you try your best to incorporate into your own teaching. Give one or two examples of situations where you have been able to motivate and enthuse a group of students about a given topic. Mention as a conclusion that you get good feedback from your teaching sessions and state briefly what people appreciate about your teaching.

9.4 How do you know that you are a good teacher?

Many candidates often rush to list the skills and attributes that make them a good teacher (i.e. basically, they answer the previous question instead: "What are the qualities of a good teacher?"). This question is not about whether you are good but about how you *know* that you are good. There are many ways in which you may know that you are good, including:

- Positive feedback from colleagues. The feedback could come either from a form that you distribute after each of your sessions, from formal feedback at appraisals (360-degree feedback or MSF – multi-source feedback)

- Being asked to become an instructor on an ALS course (or other similar course)

- Being re-invited to teach at a course (thus indicating that the first time was successful)

- Objective measures of success such as colleagues passing their exams as a result of your teaching

- Visible improvements on the shop floor, for example a junior becoming much more efficient and safer doing a procedure that you taught him

- The way in which your students interact with you during teaching sessions, i.e. the interest they pay to the topic.

When you deliver your answer, do not simply list some or all of the above. Each time you bring up a point, illustrate it with experience. For example, do not just state that your feedback was positive. Describe what the feedback was (stick to the positive feedback). If you have been re-invited to teach at a course, explain why this was the case. What did they like about you the first time round?

9.5   Which methods of teaching do you know?

This question is not too difficult but, again, the difficulty is in making it sound interesting and personal. Most candidates limit themselves to listing a few teaching methods they have come across without feeling the need to expand. The marking scheme will reward candidates who show an awareness of different teaching methods, their advantages and disadvantages, and who relate their answer to their own personal experience.

Present a broad spectrum of methods

The question is asking about the teaching methods that you *know*, not just those which you *use*. Make sure that you present not only the methods that you have encountered or used yourself, but also other methods which you may not have come across. For example, most people know about the existence of Problem-Based Learning (PBL) but have not necessarily experienced it first-hand because it is not widespread outside the confines of some medical schools.

Expand on each method

The interviewers will be looking for awareness and understanding of the different methods. In your answer, you should therefore present not only your own experience of these methods (to the extent that you have any) but also what you know of the pros and cons of each method. No need to go into massive detail: a brief explanation will suffice.

The different teaching methods

There is a wide array of teaching methods. I have set out below those which you may encounter more commonly:

One-to-one interactive teaching
- Pros: you can tailor the teaching to the needs, strengths and weaknesses of the student. It encourages maximum participation from the student and therefore optimises the learning experience. One-to-one teaching also offers flexibility because there is only one person to worry about.

- Cons: It is time-consuming and the student does not have the opportunity to learn from listening or watching his/her peers.

Small group interactive teaching (workshops, tutorials)
- Pros: interaction between different group members can raise the quality of the teaching (i.e. students feed off one another). The teaching can benefit from the experience of the various students rather than just one. It is easy to gauge

the mood and understanding of the group and for the teacher to deviate from the prepared material if there is a need to do so during the session. One particular type of teaching is known as Interprofessional Learning (IPL). This is defined as learning with, from and about other professionals (e.g. doctors and pharmacists) to improve collaboration in practice and quality of care for the patient (Centre for Advancement of Interprofessional Education - www.caipe.org.uk).

- Cons: if the group is not homogeneous, some members may feel that they are struggling whilst others may feel that they are not being stretched enough. If you are teaching a group of individuals, it is therefore important that you enquire beforehand about their level of knowledge and, if possible, that you circulate material so that those who have lesser knowledge are able to raise their game before the teaching session. This is particularly important for IPL where the students need to be at the same level (e.g. similar clinical exposure if undergraduate) and secure in their professional identities.

Formal (didactic) lectures
- Pros: you can reach a big audience quickly.
- Cons: the communication is mostly one-way. It can be difficult to give everyone in the group what they expect from the lecture. The structure is usually fairly rigid and there is limited allowance for questions and interaction. It is difficult for the lecturer to gauge the level of understanding of the students, which may result in loss of attention. Many people rely on very poor slide presentations.

Computer-based teaching (CBT)/ E-learning
- Pros: the student can take the modules at his own pace and can undertake the teaching at a time when he is the most receptive. CBT can also enable learning by repetition without boring the teacher. It is also possible to learn at a distance, even internationally.
- Cons: only works if well structured, since the student has no opportunity to address a human being.

Within each of the above settings, there are different ways of delivering teaching such as:

- Interactive discussion
- Practical simulation
- Role play
- Observation followed by repeated practice under assisted supervision and silent supervision (e.g. to learn clinical procedures)
- Problem-based learning (these days increasingly used at medical school: see next question for full details)
- Lecture followed by assessment.

9.6 What is Problem-Based Learning (PBL)? What are its pros and cons?

Problem-based learning is a teaching method based on a small group of students (typically six to ten), who are working together with the help of a tutor. The process is best described by the Maastricht "seven jump" process, *BMJ ABC of learning and teaching in medicine: Problem based learning* (2003), as follows:

Step 1	Identify and clarify unfamiliar terms presented in the scenario; the "scribe" lists those that remain unexplained after discussion
Step 2	Define the problem or problems to be discussed; students may have different views on the issues, but all should be considered; scribe records a list of agreed problems
Step 3	"Brainstorming" session to discuss the problem(s), suggesting possible explanations on basis of prior knowledge; students draw on each other's knowledge and identify areas of incomplete knowledge; scribe records all discussion
Step 4	Review steps 2 and 3 and arrange explanations into tentative solutions; scribe organises the explanations and restructures if necessary
Step 5	Formulate learning objectives; group reaches consensus on the learning objectives; tutor ensures learning objectives are focused, achievable, comprehensive, and appropriate
Step 6	Private study (all students gather information related to each learning objective)
Step 7	Group shares results of private study (students identify their learning resources and share their results); tutor checks learning and may assess the group

In PBL, the tutor is a facilitator (and not necessarily a doctor or clinician), i.e. he does not participate actively in the discussions. He is there to motivate and guide the team, helping it define and reach its objectives. This is in stark contrast to the traditional teaching methods, where the teacher has a very active role. In PBL, students are discovering for themselves, under remote supervision and guidance.

Advantages of PBL

- It is a flexible way of learning, doing away with the rigidity of traditional lectures.

- Being self-directed, students think for themselves and discover the information by themselves. This tends to lead to better retention.

- PBL does not simply promote learning the topic. It encourages students to develop other skills such as problem solving (they are confronted by a problem they have never faced before), communication (they need to argue their case to the rest of the team) and teamwork (regardless of personal opinions, it is the team as a whole which needs to resolve the problem).

- PBL allows students to make mistakes and to learn from them (the worst that can happen is wasting time). This may create broader-minded and more adventurous individuals, who can simultaneously adopt a reflective approach and do not hesitate to ask for help.

- PBL promotes initiative, focus on specific goals and research.

- Because the learning is problem-based, PBL is good at helping students place problems in the overall perspective and from a practical point of view. Students are not just learning information which could be useful to them in the future; the scenario actually shows them how the information and knowledge could be used in a concrete situation.

Disadvantages of PBL

- PBL calls for more resources than traditional teaching methods because the groups cannot be too large.

- The preparation that the tutor needs to undertake can be extensive. For example, he may need to prepare extensive reading lists and web-based resources. The tutor may also need to make himself available outside of the normal workshops in case queries arise.

- Many students are not used to PBL and may feel disorientated when confronted with such an unfamiliar method. This can be stressful.

- PBL relies on good teamwork and therefore may not function well in less homogenous groups (e.g. if one of the team does not contribute).

- If not facilitated properly, the group may easily diverge and waste time.

- The information accumulated by students is the result of their research. There is a danger that students retain information which either they do not need to know or which is too advanced for their level.

9.7 You have been asked to organise a weekly educational meeting for your colleagues. How would you approach this task?

Many of the doctors who have been asked this question and with whom I have talked have found it difficult to answer because they had "never organised a meeting before". In reality, if you think carefully about the skills that are being tested and use your logic, you should be able to provide a complete answer without much of a problem.

What is this question about?

As mentioned, this question is about your organisational skills, i.e. your ability to manage resources, time and information appropriately. It is also about your ability to work with others and communicate appropriately to achieve a positive outcome.

If you have never organised such meetings, think logically about what this would involve. Much of the content can be derived using common sense. Think about the type of meeting that you would like to be invited to:

- what would you like to learn?

- Who would you like to hear from?

- What is your objective? To organise a meeting that people will want to go to (otherwise you are wasting your time).

- It is a weekly meeting. You will need to make sure that your colleagues want to attend every week. To achieve this, you will need to organise events of quality and make participants feel involved. You cannot achieve this without ensuring that you understand what your colleagues are expecting from the educational meetings.

- If it is a weekly meeting, you cannot do all the work by yourself. You will need to arrange for different speakers; you will need to get the logistics sorted out (booking a room, photocopying the handouts, drinks, maybe sponsorship). All this takes time and you will need to get help from someone.

- You will need to make sure people can attend; therefore your meeting will need to be at a convenient time.

Much of your success will depend on your ability to communicate and work with others. You should therefore make sure that this is explicit in your answer.

Structuring the answer to the question

There are many ways in which you can structure your answer. Here is a suggestion:

Defining the meeting

- Because it is a weekly meeting you will need to find new topics every week as well as new presenters. In order to ensure the success of your project and to ensure that your colleagues get as much as they can out of the meetings, you will need to approach them and ask them what type of topics would interest them, when is the most suitable time for them and whether there are topics that they may wish to present themselves. This can be done either face to face or via a simple questionnaire that they can complete.

- Subjects can include:
    - Topics on the ST curriculum
    - Topics defined by available local speakers
    - Topics on the previous timetable
    - Risk management/patient safety
    - Journal club
    - Case of the week
    - Medical management/leadership
    - Quality improvement.

- You will also probably need to involve some of your senior colleagues who may have their own ideas about what can be achieved through these meetings. They may also have ideas that would make your life easier.

- Once you have gathered some basic information about the type of topics your colleagues want to discuss and what your seniors are aiming for, you can start putting together a document that summarises your findings and that you can discuss with your consultant. The two of you can then settle on a format and an appropriate time.

- You may also wish to discuss with your seniors whether you should limit the meeting to your immediate colleagues or whether it should be open to other departments, and even other professions (nurses, secretaries, etc.) in the team.

Sorting out the practicalities

- Once the meeting has some shape, you will need to ensure that people can attend it. You should probably have a discussion with the rota manager so that they can ensure that the time is protected and that all bleeps are covered appropriately.

- You should also liaise with a secretary to ensure that the meeting is advertised appropriately, that a room is booked and that all speakers have been notified of their engagement.

- You should be in touch with the speakers regularly to ensure that they are on track (otherwise you will have no meeting) and to arrange for any material to be given in advance (using the secretary for photocopying).

Running the meeting

- Ensure that the meeting is chaired appropriately, either by you or by someone else.

- Make sure you know how to use the computer and projector (if used) as this is the easiest way for things to fail.

- Ensure that the session is well paced so that the meeting is not too rushed or too slow.

- Ensure that those who attend have opportunities to ask questions so that they fully benefit from the meeting.

Learn from the experience & improve

- Collect feedback at the end so that you can improve from one session to the next. Remember to include space for free text:
    - What went well (and why)?
    - What should we do differently next time?

9.8 Tell us about the feedback that you have received for your teaching

Aim of the question

The aim of the question is not just to see whether you are any good at teaching (the interviewers will need to take your word for it). The question also aims to determine whether you have any insight into your own strengths and weaknesses, and whether you are able to build on the feedback that you receive and improve as a result of action taken.

The question does not explicitly state whether you should limit your answer to the positive feedback or also discuss the negative feedback that you have received. However, the marking scheme will definitely require both to be presented and you should therefore do so without waiting to be prompted.

Getting the positive-negative balance right

Whenever you face a question asking you for both positive and negative aspects of yourself, you should aim to present slightly more positive points than negative. Here you ought to aim at two or three positive points against one negative point. There are two reasons for this:

- You obviously want to emphasise your strengths more than your weaknesses.

- When talking about the negative feedback, you will need to spend time explaining how you learnt from it. This will take time. Overall, you will find that discussing one weakness will take as much time as discussing two strengths.

The positive points should come first, followed by the negative point. This has the advantage of enabling you to start the answer in an enthusiastic manner, and to conclude it with the reflective part of the negative feedback which will leave an impression of maturity. Starting with the negative point without setting out a positive context will leave a gloomy impression.

Example of an effective answer

"The feedback that I have obtained from colleagues and students has always been very positive and encouraging. One of the points, which people often mention, is that my teaching sessions are well structured and that, as a result, I am able to maintain the audience's attention for long periods of time. Medical students also very much appreciate the attention that I pay to making my sessions interactive. They have found that they retained the information much more and many of them have actually obtained good results in their finals as a result.

On the less positive side, there was a specific workshop for which I had not anticipated the diversity of backgrounds the students came from and, in particular, I had not taken account of the fact that half of them had already had experience of the specialty, whilst the other half had not. At the time this caused some problems with comprehension.

Since this particular incident, I take much greater care to discuss with the students before the session what they know and what they seek to gain from the session, and I have not had any more issues."

This answer is effective because:

- There is a good balance between positive and negative. The two paragraphs are of equal length.

- The negative feedback is well presented, with an element of personal reflection, which emphasises the candidate's willingness to learn.

- The negative feedback is specific and refers to a temporary error of judgement rather than lasting incompetence. It has also been remedied.

Example of an effective answer (partial – negative paragraph only)

"… As far as negative feedback is concerned, there have been a couple of occasions where people commented on the fact that my slides were too wordy. It is an issue which I think is quite common and to resolve this I attended a presentation skills course at the Royal College, as a result of which I have learnt to make better use of pictures and diagrams. I have also become more conscious of the fact that you don't need to put everything down on your slides and that it can be just as effective to address the audience directly, with the slide showing just the key headings. It makes the speaker more engaging."

9.9 Tell us about a bad (or your worst) teaching experience that you have had as a teacher (i.e. not as a delegate)

Whether you are asked about a bad or your worst teaching experience makes no difference at all. As always, when asked about something negative, you will be expected to explain how you have dealt with it and how you learnt from it; therefore, what matters more is that you choose an experience that enables you to sell yourself effectively.

Examples you can mention

Since the emphasis is on the reflective process, you should choose an example which has potential for this. This may include situations where:

- your teaching session was too complicated or too easy for your audience

- your audience was made up of people who had very varied backgrounds

- you had to deal with disruptive students in your audience

- you failed to prepare adequately (e.g. unable to answer questions)

- one of your trainees consistently failed to understand what you were trying to teach them and you struggled through multiple alternatives.

Note that you don't have to mention your *actual* worst experience if you really messed up. No one will know what the truth is. Simply choose any negative experience on which you reflected meaningfully.

Structuring your answer

To answer this question, you can follow the STAR structure:

Situation/Task	Explain what type of teaching session it was and why it went wrong
Action	Demonstrate the initiative that you used at the time to correct the problem. How did you communicate? How did you alter your plans to adapt to the changing circumstance?
Result/Reflect	What happened at the end? What did you learn from the situation? How has it helped you improve your teaching abilities?

9.10 What is clinical audit?

With this question, the interviewers will be testing your understanding of the audit process and therefore you will need to go well beyond giving out a simple definition. They will be expecting you to raise two points:

- A clear explanation of what an audit is, i.e. a definition in your own words
- A description of the audit cycle.

Definition of clinical audit

There are several definitions of clinical audit, some of which date back to 1989 and 1983. However, the most recent is that published in *Principles for Best Practice in Clinical Audit* (2002) by the National Institute for Health and Clinical Excellence (NICE):

"Clinical audit is a quality improvement process that seeks to improve patient care and outcomes through systematic review of care against explicit criteria and the review of change. Aspects of the structure, process and outcome of care are selected and systematically evaluated against explicit criteria. Where indicated, changes are implemented at an individual, team, or service level and further monitoring is used to confirm improvement in healthcare delivery."

At an interview, beware of trying to regurgitate definitions. Most are lengthy, use words which are not natural to you, and sometimes are deliberately vague to cover wide areas. Your task is therefore to transform this definition into something more easily digestible. For example:

"Clinical audit is a review of current health practices against agreed standards, designed to ensure that, as clinicians, we provide the best level of care to our patients and that we constantly seek to improve our practice where it is not matching those standards"

or

"Audits are a systematic examination of current practice to assess how well an institution or a practitioner is performing against set standards. Essentially it is a method for systematically reflecting on, reviewing and improving practice."

The audit cycle

Some of the marks for this question will relate to your understanding of the audit cycle. Make sure that you can discuss each of the following steps without hesitation:

Step 1: Identify an issue or problem

The aim of an audit is to ensure that your clinical practice is in line with best practice. Doctors should continually audit their practice, ideally doing frequent rapid audits (e.g. the last five patients with diabetic ketoacidosis) and making changes. This is much more useful than a larger audit as it is unlikely that there will be many more learning points from reviewing 100 patients than from reviewing five, and the benefit still comes from improving the system and re-auditing it. Primary target topics for audits may include:

- Any area of clinical practice where problems have arisen; this could have been identified through a rising level of complaints, the occurrence or recurrence of mistakes.
- The need to check compliance with national guidelines.
- Areas of clinical practice where there are clear risks either because they deal with a high volume of patients or because there are high costs associated with these procedures/practices.
- Any obvious areas where improvements can be brought in (often identified through observation or experience).

Step 2: Identify a standard

Clinical practice will be assessed against a standard which needs to be defined at the outset. Standards should be drawn from the best available evidence and in many cases are set by NICE, the relevant Royal Colleges, or other specialty-related associations (e.g. British Orthopaedics Association). When standards are not readily available, a Trust may define its own local standards. A Trust may also want to impose on itself standards which are more stringent than those available.

Step 3: Collect data on current practice

The data should be collected in respect of a pre-agreed period of clinical practice (e.g. period between date 1 and date 2) for a specific group of individuals (e.g. all asymptomatic patients who presented to clinic for the first time). These criteria will have been agreed at the outset. In collecting data, care should be taken to ensure that any patient identifiable data is removed.

Note that there are clinical audit departments in hospitals that exist to support your audits! As such, they will help design pro formas, collect notes, possibly even do any statistical analysis required, and then help present the data. The important thing is to start early and communicate with them.

Step 4: Assess conformity of clinical practice with the standard

Once the data has been summarised and analysed, the result is compared to the standard to determine how well it has been met.

More importantly, if the standard is not met, the reasons for non-compliance should be identified so that they can be remedied. Although identifying non-compliance is relatively easy, identifying why there is a problem may take more time. In some cases, it may be necessary to carry out a study of the problem to understand the causes of the underperformance.

Step 5: Implementing change

This is the step that justifies the whole process i.e. improving practice so that the standard is matched. Examples of changes may include:

- Altering protocols (especially simplifying them)
- Reorganising service, altering roles and responsibilities
- Providing further training to key staff
- Raising awareness of guidelines with staff (e.g. regular teaching sessions, creation of an intranet)
- Improving documentation
- Altering a labelling system
- Changing equipment.

Step 6: Closing the loop: re-audit

Once all changes have been implemented, the dust should be allowed to settle. After an agreed period of time, once the changes have had a chance to have an impact on clinical practice, clinical practice should be audited again to measure their impact. To be effective and meaningful, a re-audit should use the same sample, methods and data analysis. Hopefully, the re-audit will show that the standard has been matched. If not, further changes will be required and further re-audits should be carried out.

Carrying out the re-audit is commonly referred to as "closing the loop" or "completing the audit cycle". This is by far the weakest point of the process, partly because of turnover of staff and partly because the process of audit still remains poorly understood.

Note: it may be that, in the meantime, the standard has changed (e.g. in view of new research). In this case, the re-audit will constitute a new audit and it can be referred to as the "audit spiral".

9.11　Tell us about an interesting audit that you did

Structuring your answer

This question is designed to test your understanding of the audit process/cycle through the description of one example. To demonstrate that you understand clearly the principles of audits, you should therefore aim to address explicitly the following points:

- *Why the audit was deemed necessary* (i.e. what was the problem which led to the initiation of an audit?).

- *The standard used.* Typically this would be guidelines from a Royal College or some other association; but it may be that you had to derive your own standard by doing a literature search for example. If this is the case, be sure to mention it.

- *The result of the audit,* i.e. did clinical practice match the standard and if not, why not?

- *What proposals for change you made and which were implemented*

- *Whether you did a re-audit or not.* If you did not do the re-audit (which will be the case for the vast majority of candidates), make sure that you demonstrate your understanding of this crucial step by saying something such as "Since this was the end of my attachment, I did not have time to be involved in the re-audit, but we planned it for 6 months down the line". If you have taken the trouble to check the results of the re-audit with the local team then this would be to your credit, because it would demonstrate the effectiveness of the changes that you had proposed and implemented.

  Consider doing a re-audit as your audit. This will save all the planning and thinking and show that you understand the process. Even better, start with a re-audit (doing just five sets of notes), make changes to the system as needed and audit again with another five case records.

- *What your role was* (i.e. initiated, devised a pro forma, collected the data, analysed, discussed with senior colleagues, identified ideas for change, wrote report, presented to local team/audit meeting).

- *Presentation/Publication.* If the audit was presented outside the local environment, or even published either as such or as an abstract, make sure that you mention it.

Choosing an "interesting" audit

The question uses the word "interesting". However, it is possible that the audit which you personally enjoyed the most is not the audit which will help you score the most points.

Your main criterion for the choice of an example should be the extent of your involvement in the project and the strength/complexity of the audit, as these are the factors that will influence the marking the most.

If you can, focus on an audit which is relevant to the specialty to which you are applying. Not only might some marks be allocated for the relevance of the example to the specialty, but, even if this is not the case, the interviewers will be naturally drawn towards an example which they can relate to. Of course, if you find that you have no specialty-related audits which are of any interest but that another audit would make a far more powerful answer then use the latter.

Concluding your answer

The use of the word "interesting" in the question means that you really ought to explain why you feel that the particular audit you have just described is "interesting". It could be because of the topic itself, or because of the potential for change that it offered. It may also be because it gave you an opportunity to develop new skills such as delegation and management, and perhaps IT too. Whatever your reasons, make sure that you explain them (albeit succinctly).

You may also emphasise how much this experience taught you about the audit process and how it gave you an impetus to become involved in other audit projects. You can then name a project in which you are currently involved (name, not describe, otherwise it will take too long).

9.12 Tell us about your audit experience

How this question is marked

The marking schemes for this question vary widely between deaneries, specialties and grades. Some deaneries will simply assess on the number and quality of the audits that candidates have done, whilst others will use much more complex criteria, even at the most junior levels. Since you will not have access to the marking scheme before you answer the question, include as much information as possible in your answer. With this question, the interviewers will assess you on the following criteria:

- *The number of audits* in which you have been involved. This will be judged in relation to the expectation at your level. Most junior doctors are expected to complete one audit per post or at least two a year.

- *Your role in the audit process*. If you have been involved simply in collecting data then you are most likely to score less than if you have initiated and/or led an audit. Doing audits with one or two others allows you to complete more in the time!

- *The complexity of your audits*. You will need to explain what the audits were about and what standards you were testing clinical practice against. A minor audit will impress less than a complex audit. Not all deaneries allocate marks to complexity, but those that don't still account for it subconsciously because the answer will sound more impressive if the audits are complex. Any audit that makes a change and is then re-audited will score well, however simple.

- *The usefulness of your audits*, i.e. the extent to which they identified variation from the standard and led to change. Some deaneries allocate extra marks to candidates who have formed evidence-based guidelines as a result of their audits.

- *Whether you understand the audit process/cycle*

- *Whether or not you completed the loop*. This is unlikely to be relevant for most trainees, as many of you will have moved on before you could perform a re-audit. Nevertheless, some deaneries allocate marks for this.

- *Whether the audit results were presented* and at what level (i.e. just local, or regional, or even national)? Some marking schemes provide further marks for abstracts.

In order to prepare for this question, you would therefore be well advised to draw a list of your audits and to establish for each of them whether you can gain marks in any of the above categories.

Delivering your answer

If you have done more than two audits, you can introduce your overall experience with a sentence of the type:

"I have carried out five audits over the past 4 years, including three which I led personally from initiation to conclusion. Two of these audits were extremely useful in improving clinical care."

or

"Over the past 4 years, I have conducted five audits, including three which are specifically related to <specialty that you are applying for>. The most interesting audits were ..."

You would then develop the two audits in question in line with the marking criteria set out on the previous page and the structure set out in 9.11.

If you have done one or two audits, then you can simply take them one by one, ensuring that you limit yourself to a total time of 2 minutes. Simply detail your experience using the points described in the previous section.

If you have not completed an audit but you have been partially involved, be honest about it but do not make a negative judgement on your experience such as "Unfortunately my audit experience is very poor because I did not have the opportunity to be involved". Not only does this tell the interviewers how they should interpret your lack of experience (i.e. negatively), it also does not present you as a proactive individual who seeks the experience he/she needs. Simply concentrate on the facts, explain whatever you have been involved with and how this has given you a better understanding of the audit process (see 9.10 for more detail).

If you have done no audit at all then you probably won't score anything but you might as well try to gain some credit by explaining your understanding of the audit process, trying to relate it to your own experience (see 9.10), which you might have gained by attending departmental clinical governance meetings or training sessions. At least say you are currently planning one with the clinical audit department and will start next week.

9.13 Why are audits important?

This question is very factual and, unless you have reflected on the audit process by yourself, you will simply need to learn a few lines to make sure that you provide a sensible answer.

Here are some of the key benefits of audit:

- As one of the key pillars of clinical governance, audit ensures that quality of care is maintained at an agreed standard. It enables the identification of problems and, through the audit cycle, ensures that solutions are implemented until the desired standard of care is reached.

- Audit encourages services to make better use of resources and therefore become more efficient

- The data gathered during the audit process can be used:

  - To inform patients about the standard of care that they receive (following a range of new reforms, including the emphasis on patient choice, providing information to patients has become a key priority)
  - To feed the appraisal and assessment process which forms a key part of the new revalidation process
  - To demonstrate to your Trust, its managers and other authorities that you are working efficiently and providing a quality service. This will encourage them to help you develop the service further.
  - To share information with other Trusts on local practices and their efficacy in meeting standards and providing quality care.

- The audit process is a good exercise to train and develop juniors. In an era where the training of doctors in management is often criticised, audits offer a good platform to learn about service improvement and quality of service provision.

9.14 What are the problems associated with the audit process?

To answer this question well, you may wish to distinguish between problems associated with audits generally and problems associated with audits carried out by junior doctors (in fact, some deaneries ask about the problems associated with junior doctors' audits).

If you have done one or more audits yourself, you must have identified at least one or two of the problems listed below. In delivering your answer, feel free to use your own audit experience to illustrate your answer in order to give it a more personal, less didactic, slant.

Problems associated with audit generally

- Audits are most often a local process. Though they are useful at improving local practice, they may not be so transferable to other Trusts or units. Other Trusts may not be able to replicate the same approach and, if similar problems are identified, the resolution methods which worked well in one Trust may not achieve the same results when applied in a different Trust.

- Audits are often based on retrospective data (usually patient notes). The data available in the notes was not collected for the specific purpose of the audit. Therefore there may be discrepancies in the way it was recorded and, in some cases, the data may be missing.

- Audits identify that there is a problem or a lack of compliance with a given standard; identifying a solution to the problem identified may not be so easy. Further studies may be required, which can be lengthy.

- Although there are audit departments in most Trusts, those who actually carry out the audits are most often the clinicians, who have many other responsibilities and therefore may not focus entirely on the process. They are also often inexperienced in that activity. This may lead to delay in the implementation of change.

- Unless there is a strong departmental policy of rationalisation of the audit process, topics are not always chosen in the order of priority. This may mean that important areas are neglected, whilst clinicians take on audits which are affordable in terms of resources and are less time-consuming.

The following two points are problems associated with the consequences of the audit process (though not specifically about the audit process itself):

- Audits may identify that non-compliance is linked with the under-performance of specific members of the team or the criticism of certain practices. This makes audit a useful tool, but may also lead to the demotivation of parts of the team if some people feel more targeted than others.

- One of the outcomes of audit is the implementation of change in order to improve standards of care. This change may lead to resistance from some members of the team.

These problems are particularly acute when audits are conducted across boundaries, e.g. the transfer of patients, post cardiac surgery, from the intensive care unit back to the ward. It is easy to criticise another team (e.g. their discharge summaries), but is difficult to change and can in fact inflame the situation. The way to overcome this is to jointly audit the patient's pathway and keep the focus on what is best for the patient.

Problems associated with audits being carried out by junior doctors

- Junior doctors rotate frequently and, if they are around long enough to carry out an audit, they are most likely to leave before a re-audit can be performed. From their own perspective, they are unable to see the impact of the changes that they have helped introduce. From the departmental perspective, it may be more difficult to find someone to do the re-audit (less glamorous, and they would not benefit from the input of the junior who originally carried out the audit).

- In some cases, the audit analysis is either not completed or the recommendations are not taken to implementation stage, thus defeating the whole purpose of the exercise.

- Junior doctors may not command the respect that seniors would have. They may find it more difficult to obtain data or gain support for their audit project.

- Junior doctors tend to choose audit topics which are easier and take shorter periods of time. These topics may not be aligned with departmental strategy or may not be of great importance in the overall scale of things (i.e. the audit is a box-ticking exercise to look good on the CV).

9.15 What is the difference between audit and research?

This is a question that most candidates have heard about and the interviewers know it. There is therefore no excuse for being unprepared. If you have been involved in audit and research activities then you will be able to draw upon your experience to illustrate your answers.

The fundamental difference

The term "audit" is often confused by clinicians, who describe as "audits" projects that are actually research projects. This is fairly common on CVs and application forms, which is why they are keen to test your understanding at the interview. Your application form and CV will be reviewed at the portfolio station. There is nothing more embarrassing than to describe perfectly the difference between audit and research, only to discover that your own documents contradict your words.

Audit is a process which compares clinical practice against set standards, i.e. you are simply trying to determine whether your practice matches the level of care expected of you. Are you following the established guidelines or your own guidelines? Are you aligned with best practice? How much variability is there within your care processes? Are you a learning organisation? Are you doing what you think you are doing?

Research does not check whether you are complying with standards. Instead, its aim is to create new knowledge that can then be used to develop new standards of care. Research determines whether new treatments work and to what extent they do. It is also used to determine which treatments are better than others so that appropriate recommendations can be made.

So, essentially, research helps establish best practice whilst audit checks that best practice is being applied in practice.

Examples

If you are trying to establish
- whether x, y and z are correctly recorded in patients' notes; or
- whether test X is being offered to a specific type of patients, or;
- that the complication rate for a specific procedure is less or equal to the percentage specified in the XYZ Association guidelines,

then this is an audit because you are trying to establish that your current practice is in line with what would be expected.

If, on the other hand, you are trying to establish

- whether procedure A gives better outcomes than procedure B; or
- whether sending patients advance information improves the take-up rate of a specific procedure; or
- whether systematic hand washing decreases infection rate,

then it is research, because you are trying to discover new information, which may then be used to implement new guidelines.

Other differences

- Research is based on a hypothesis, whereas audit measures compliance against standards.

- Research is theory-driven and a one-off process. Audit is practice-driven and a continuous process.

- Results from research can be generalised. Audit results are mostly relevant locally.

- Research is not always conducted by those involved in service provision. Audits most often are.

- Research may involve experimentation, whereas audits never involve experimentation. Audits are mostly a data-gathering exercise.

- Research may involve trying out new treatments, whereas audits never involve new treatments or interference with the management of the patient.

- Research involves strict selection of candidates, allocating these candidates between different treatment groups and validating sample size. In audit, the sample of patients used is not put together scientifically, sample size is not validated and patients are never placed into different treatment groups.

- Research requires ethical approval. Audits rarely do (ethical issues in audit mainly revolve around confidentiality or collection of that data).

Many audits morph into pseudo-research where lots of data is collected and a new pro forma is designed, but in such cases there is no gold standard, no change to the service and often no uptake or spread within the department (particularly after the enthusiast has left).

9.16 Tell us about your research experience

This question can be asked in all specialties and at all grades, even at grades where many candidates are unlikely to have had any substantial involvement in research. There are easy ways to score points, even if your experience is limited.

The boxes you need to tick

Though the question asks for your experience and nothing more specific, most marking schedules will in fact include much more than that. In order to provide an answer which is as complete as possible, you will need to address the following points:

- The number, type and quality of research projects undertaken.
- The outcomes of projects, including publications and presentations.
- Your role, including any experience of recruiting patients, seeking ethical approval or grant applications.
- Research-related skills that you gained from your experience, e.g. literature review, critical appraisal, statistics and general understanding of research principles.
- General skills gained from your experience, e.g. writing skills, negotiation, communication, teamwork, planning, time management, etc.
- Any relevant courses attended such as research methodology, critical appraisal or statistics courses.
- Your future plans with regard to research.

Answering the question

- *If you have substantial research experience*, you will not have the time to describe all of it. You should aim to summarise the extent of your experience first "I have been involved in four research projects including one randomised controlled trial, two studies and one national trial over the past four years as part of the PhD that I am currently completing". You could then summarise one or two of your projects (those you are most proud of) before discussing the extent of your publications and presentations. End the answer by mentioning the courses that you attended and discussing your future research aims and interests.

- *If you have been involved in a small number of research projects*, describe each project briefly, setting out your role, the courses you attended, the publications and presentations which originated from your experience and the skills that you gained, as well as your future research aims and interests.

- **If you have no research experience at all**, think carefully first about any project in which you have been involved and which is <u>not</u> an audit. Can this project be considered research, even if it was informal? If yes, then you can present whatever you did in line with the principles explained so far. If not, then don't panic. Many people will be in your situation and you can still score marks by mentioning some of the following:

  - Literature reviews undertaken (which gave you an insight into research principles)

  - Case reports published. Strictly-speaking, case reports do not constitute research because they are simply reporting how a specific patient presented or was managed. However, by sharing your experience with others, you are helping them change or improve their practice. Other benefits include the literature search you will have completed, the rigour of having to write concisely and the overall experience of how to construct a paper and bibliography. Case reports are part of the pool of evidence used in evidence-based medicine and therefore they are relevant to the "spirit" of the question. Some marking schemes make specific allowance for case reports, so make sure you mention yours

  - Attendance at journal clubs (which will have given you critical appraisal skills and an understanding of the research process)

  - Attendance at conferences (where you have gained an appreciation of research methodologies)

  - Research-related courses.

9.17 Why is research important?

Fundamental importance of research – the overall perspective

Essentially, the aim of research is to drive medical advancement by developing a pool of knowledge which can then be translated into better patient care. Research therefore can benefit patients directly through improved treatments and procedures. Translation of the key messages from the literature to routine medical practice is, however, very slow.

Importance of research to a Trust

- The Trust's reputation may be enhanced. Not only might this attract more patients (and therefore more income), but also higher quality staff and more trainees.

- A Trust involved in research through clinical trials can provide some of its patients with early access to the latest technologies for diagnosing and treating disease.

Importance of research to a junior doctor

- It enables them to understand the evidence on which decisions are based. In particular the treatments and procedures they are using in their everyday practice would have greater meaning to them.

- Nurturing a practice founded on evidence-based medicine (EBM - see 9.20) involves an ability to critically appraise current medical evidence. Having an insight into what constitutes good and bad research as well as the structure of levels of medical evidence and statistical concepts is an excellent basis to develop EBM for the future. This can be gained by undertaking research or even, more simply, by attending journal clubs.

- Since medical practice is constantly evolving, it is essential to keep up to date with current published research. This is one component of continuous professional development (CPD).

- A good grounding and insight into the ethics and procedures of medical research is important. Many trainees will have future roles in experimental therapies or managing patients who may be involved in clinical trials.

- Advances in medicine are inextricably linked to research and giving trainee doctors inspiration at an early stage may encourage further advancements in the future.

- It provides a good insight into a specialty and often leads to career progression within that field, even if that had not been the previous intention.

- It enables them to gain a number of skills such as organisational skills (working to deadlines, organising data, planning a project, notation, integrity, etc.) and writing and presentation skills.

Delivering the answer

If you have been involved in research, make sure that you illustrate the above points with some of your experience. If you have limited experience of research, then you can simply hold an intelligent discussion using some of the above points.

9.18 Do you think that all trainees should do research?

Interpreting the question

This question is often misunderstood. Many candidates say, "Yes everyone should do research because research is important". There is no doubt that research is important but it does not mean that everyone <u>has</u> to be involved in it. In popular specialties, research is often done to develop a competitive advantage over peers. This is again a poor reason for doing it.

With this question, the interviewers are testing:

- Your understanding of the pros and cons of undertaking research at a junior level
- Your appreciation of the importance of research to a junior doctor (which we have addressed in 9.17).

Key points:

- If "research" means time out being taken to undertake a PhD, MD, MPhil, or other degree, then it is probably not necessary for all trainees to become involved. The reasons for this are that:

  - A lot of research achieves little and/or does not get published.
  - Many research projects do not get completed through lack of time or lack of funding.
  - The limited funding and resources are best saved for those with real enthusiasm or ability.
  - Some trainees may not particularly like research. Making such a big commitment might demotivate them and be counterproductive.
  - Taking time out to do research means moving away from clinical duties and therefore creating greater difficulties in continuing clinical training. If the research period is too great, there is a danger of deskilling.
  - Formal research is probably best left to those who enjoy it and feel that they can fruitfully contribute. In fact MMC recognises this by creating special academic posts for those who want to develop a research interest. The system therefore recognises that not everyone needs to have a formal research interest.

- Even if they are not formally involved in research, trainees need to understand the principles of research in order to be safe and effective clinicians. In the context of evidence-based practice, trainees will need to understand how research is conducted, and what makes bad and good research. They will need to be able to critically analyse papers in order to determine their validity and how the findings can be interpreted to help clinical decision makings (for more details, see 9.17 – paragraph on the importance of research to junior doctors). Although first-hand research experience would be useful to gain such understanding, it can also be gained through other means, such as:

- Attending journal clubs
- Attending conferences and relevant courses (statistics, critical appraisal, research methodologies)
- Getting involved in smaller, ad hoc or informal research projects (e.g. one afternoon per week), which will not distract from clinical training
- Doing literature searches, for example to set a standard for an audit or as part of evidence-based practice.

Answering the question

In answering this question, it is important that you debate the issue rather than rush into giving a strong opinion. There is no harm at all in having a strong opinion, but you need to ensure that it is put into perspective. You should demonstrate your understanding of research, its importance to clinicians and the issues raised by introducing research in the training curriculum.

If you have any meaningful experience of research, then make sure that you talk about it in your answer. Rather than discussing the usefulness of research to a trainee from a general perspective, you will gain marks for relating your arguments to your own experience (i.e. discussing how you benefited from your own research experience).

Similarly, if you have little research experience, but feel that you have gained appropriate competencies through other means, then you should state this, confidently.

Your experience is more valuable than any general statement.

9.19 What do you understand by the term "Research Governance"?

This question has been asked mostly at ST3 level, though a few unfortunate candidates were quizzed on it at ST1 level (e.g. Ophthalmology). Although you will not be expected to have an in-depth understanding of this concept, being able to put together an intelligent answer would set you apart.

Whenever you hear the word "governance", it refers to a set of rules that govern the way a particular activity should be undertaken. For example, clinical governance sets out the principles that doctors should follow to provide the best clinical care for their patients and continuous quality improvement.

"Research governance" is a framework of standards of good practice, applied to research. The full extent of these principles and regulations is set out in a document published in 2005 by the Department of Health: *Research Governance Framework for Health and Social Care*. This document is available from the Department of Health's website (www.doh.gov.uk. Document DH_4108962)

Key features

Ethics
- The dignity, safety, rights and wellbeing of patients should come first
- Approval of the Research and Development (R&D) Directorate and the appropriate Research Ethics Committee must be obtained before any research commences
- Informed consent should be sought. This is important for all patients, but particularly so for those who lack capacity, and when there is use of human tissue
- Patient data should be kept confidential
- Research should respect the diversity of the population in terms of age, gender, race, etc. so that the evidence available reflects society
- Any risks taken during the research must be justified in relation to the benefits of that research. Risk must always be minimised and clearly explained to the patient and the ethics committee in advance
- Research involving animals must ensure that the number of animals used is kept to a minimum and that harm to these animals is minimised. Whenever possible, the use of animals should be replaced with alternative methods

Science
- A review of current evidence should be undertaken before any research is carried out. Duplicating work is unethical, as is research which contributes little to existing knowledge
- All research proposals should be peer-reviewed

- All trials involving patients should be approved by the Medicines and Healthcare products Regulatory Agency
- Data collected should be kept to allow further analysis and monitoring by relevant authorities

Information
- Information about research carried out, including positive and negative outcomes, should be made freely available to the public in a user-friendly language. The timing of release of information needs to take account of commercial sensitivities
- Those involved in research activities should remain open to critical review through the means of publications or other appropriate ways

Health and Safety
- The safety of participants, including research staff, comes first at all times

Finance
- Full compliance with Treasury rules is required
- Organisations employing researchers should be in a position to compensate anyone harmed by the research
- Researchers should make arrangements for the management of financial and other resources provided for the study; this includes the management of any intellectual property rights

9.20 What is "Evidence-Based Medicine"?

Definition of evidence-based medicine

Evidence-based medicine (EBM) has been defined as "the conscientious, explicit, and judicious use of current best evidence in making decisions about the care of individual patients. The practice of evidence-based medicine means integrating individual clinical expertise with the best available external clinical evidence from systematic research." (David Sackett et al., *Evidence Based Medicine: What It Is and What It Isn't*, BMJ 312, no.7023 (1996))

In 2000, David Sackett revised his definition as follows: "integration of best research evidence with clinical expertise and patient values." David Sackett et al., *Evidence-Based Medicine: How to Practice and Teach EBM* (New York: Churchill Livingstone, 2000), 1

The steps involved in evidence-based medicine

- A question arises regarding the care of a particular patient.

- The physician constructs a well-defined clinical question from the case in order to resolve the problem.

- For treatments, the PICO formula can be used to make Medline searches more specific (Population, Intervention, Comparison and Outcome).

- The physician conducts a search of the existing literature by using the most appropriate resources.

- The evidence is then appraised for its validity and applicability. The physician then determines the best available evidence.

- The physician integrates the evidence with his clinical practice and the patient's preferences to find a practical solution to the original problem.

- The result is then evaluated with the patient.

Answering the question

Step 1: Define briefly what evidence-based medicine is

You should be wary of using ready-made definitions (the same applies to the classic definition of clinical governance) as they simply demonstrate your ability to regurgitate ready-made answers and do not highlight any personal understanding of the underlying issues.

The above definitions also use words that are unfamiliar to many people and which are best avoided (for example, people may not know that "judicious" means "based on sound judgement").

Try to build your own practical definition, showing that you have a good understanding of what EBM entails. EBM is essentially a combination of the best available research evidence with your own clinical expertise and judgement. This is then applied to a specific case, taking into account patient values.

Step 2: Explain the different steps involved

Step 3: If you have one, give a brief example of a situation where you used evidence-based medicine

This might include:

- Having had to deal with a patient for whom normal guidelines did not fit.
- A situation where the existing guidelines were out of date and where you needed to derive your own approach using more recent evidence.
- A situation where national guidelines were not suitable for the local pattern of disease.
- Situations where there are new, controversial treatments which are not yet in routine practice. You would then evaluate the evidence with your colleagues to devise a local strategy.
- Situations where a patient may have read about a drug in the press and may have a particular interpretation. You would need to review the evidence before presenting your personal or departmental perspective.
- Situations where you have to guide the patient to make an informed decision. This would involve presenting the relevant evidence and the efficacy, benefits and risks of the different options according to the literature.

9.21 What are the different levels of evidence available?

There are three different ways to describe the levels of evidence. The easiest classification system is:

Level	Description
Ia	Systematic review or meta-analysis of randomised controlled trials
Ib	At least one randomised controlled trial
IIa	At least one well-designed controlled study without randomisation
IIb	At least one well-designed quasi-experimental study, such as a cohort study
III	Well-designed non-experimental descriptive studies, such as comparative studies, correlation studies, case–control studies and case series
IV	Expert committee reports, opinions and/or clinical experience of respected authorities

In my experience, many candidates have learnt the above table and know it well (particularly in surgery). I would therefore encourage you to try to remember it if you can. If you struggle to remember this, particularly at interview, don't panic. It is important you remain confident and explain what you can.

A simple answer such as: "I cannot remember the exact detail of each level; however, I do know that the different levels of evidence range from the strongest level which is a systematic review all the way to the weakest which is represented by the opinion of experts", may not sound much but it is better than waffling desperately through a confused list.

9.22 In evidence-based medicine, why does a clinician need to take account of his/her own clinical expertise?

This is a question which is often asked as a follow-up to test the candidates' understanding of the fundamentals of evidence-based practice.

David Sackett (the author of the definition of clinical governance) states:

"External evidence can inform, but never replace, individual clinical expertise. [This] expertise will assist the practitioner in deciding whether the external evidence applies to the individual client at all, and, if so, how it should be integrated into the clinical decision"

Evidence-Based Medicine: How to Practice and Teach EBM (New York: Churchill Livingstone, 2000), 1

There are several reasons why evidence alone is insufficient and clinical experience matters. Here are a few:

- The study or trial that constitutes the best available evidence may not be directly relevant to the patient and may need to be adapted. For example, the patient may be in a different age range or ethnicity to those used in the study.

- There may be evidence that the administration of a given treatment has a positive impact on some patients. Judgement is needed to determine whether, for this particular patient, the benefits outweigh the risks.

- The patient may have co-morbidities which may influence the decision.

9.23 Is evidence-based medicine applicable to all specialties?

This question has come up several times in Psychiatry, though there is no reason why it could not be asked in others.

Is EBM applicable to all specialties?

The answer to this question is that evidence-based medicine is applicable to all specialties but to varying degrees. The reasons are as follows:

- **Different levels of research activities**
  Some specialties are very strong on research (either because there is more of a research culture or because research can more easily be carried out due to the sheer number and the homogeneity of the patients the specialty deals with). These specialties therefore have a greater body of evidence than others. In areas where research is lacking, the clinician needs to rely principally on his judgement to make a decision.

- **Lack of high-level evidence available**
  In some specialties, it may be difficult to find high-level evidence. By itself, this is not a problem since the clinician would then look for lower levels of evidence. However, such evidence may not be widely published.

- **Individuality of patient**
  The impact of social and environmental factors may be so strong that each decision should very much be taken at an individual level and no evidence (which is likely to be anecdotal) could be reliably used to make decisions.

- **Little historic information on older treatments**
  Some of the long-standing treatments may not be backed up by much evidence despite the fact that they are deemed to be effective. This may make it more difficult to compare their efficacy in relation to other treatments.

Answering the question

If you have an example or two (preferably from the specialty you are applying for) then use them to illustrate your answer.

9.24 Can you describe what clinical governance is?

A well-known definition that you should avoid

The most widely used definition of clinical governance is as follows:

> "A framework through which NHS organisations are accountable for continually improving the quality of their services and safeguarding high standards of care by creating an environment in which excellence in clinical care will flourish."
>
> G Scally and L J Donaldson, *Clinical governance and the drive for quality improvement in the new NHS in England,* BMJ (4 July 1998): 61-65

Although you should of course familiarise yourself with this definition, there is no need to memorise it. Under pressure, most candidates remember the beginning and the end, and mess up the middle part. Even if you remembered it perfectly, you would only demonstrate that you have a good memory and not that you understand the concept.

Instead, you should derive your own practical and down-to-earth definition.

How can you define clinical governance?

Anything which avoids the word "flourish" and can be delivered in your own natural words will do, providing it addresses the concepts of quality and accountability. Here are a few examples:

> Clinical governance is a quality assurance process, designed to ensure that standards of care are maintained and improved and that the NHS is accountable to the public.

> Clinical governance is an umbrella term that encompasses a range of activities in which clinicians should become involved in order to maintain and improve the quality of the care they provide to patients and to ensure full accountability of the system to patients.

The 7 pillars of clinical governance

Traditionally, clinical governance has been described using 7 key pillars. Although it has been refined over the past few years, this approach remains the easiest to remember and to describe at a trainee interview level. It is also the approach that your interviewers are most likely to expect from you since this is what they would have learnt too. The 7 pillars are as follows:

Clinical Effectiveness & Research

Clinical effectiveness means ensuring that everything you do is designed to provide the best outcomes for patients, i.e. that you do "the right thing to the right person at the right time in the right place". In practice, it means:

- Adopting an evidence-based approach in the management of patients
- Changing your practice: developing new protocols or guidelines based on experience and evidence if current practice is shown to be inadequate
- Implementing NICE guidelines, National Service Frameworks and other national standards to ensure optimal care (when they are not superseded by more recent and more effective treatments)
- Conducting research to develop the body of evidence available and therefore enhancing the level of care provided to patients in future.

Audit

See 9.10 for full details on clinical audit. The aim of the audit process is to ensure that clinical practice is continuously monitored and that deficiencies in relation to set standards of care are remedied.

Risk Management

Risk Management involves having robust systems in place to understand, monitor and minimise the risks to patients and staff and to learn from mistakes and near misses. When things go wrong in the delivery of care, doctors and other clinical staff should feel safe admitting it and be able to learn and share what they have learnt. This includes:

- Complying with protocols (hand washing, discarding sharps, identifying patients correctly, etc.)
- Learning from mistakes and near misses (informally for small issues, formally for the bigger events – see next point)
- Reporting any significant adverse events via critical incident forms, looking closely at complaints, etc.
- Assessing the risks identified by likelihood of recurrence and the severity of impact if an incident did occur. Implementing processes to reduce the risk and its impact (the level of implementation will often depend on the budget available and the seriousness of the risk)
- Promoting a blame-free culture to encourage everyone to report problems and mistakes.

Education & Training

50% of medical knowledge changes every 5 years and so education and training are essential for clinicians to keep up to date. Further, professional development needs to be driven by self-directed lifelong learning. In practice, for doctors this involves:

- Attending courses and conferences (commonly referred to as CPD – Continuous Professional Development)
- Taking relevant exams
- Regular workplace-based assessment, designed to ensure that doctors have the appropriate competencies
- Appraisals (which are a means of identifying and discussing weaknesses, and opportunities for personal development).

Patient and Public Involvement (PPI)

PPI ensures that the services provided are effective, that improvements are made from the patient's perspective, and that patients and the public are involved in the development of services and the monitoring of treatment outcomes. This is being implemented through a number of initiatives and organisations, including:

- Local patient feedback questionnaires
- The Patient Advice and Liaison Service (PALS): resolves patient concerns
- National patient surveys organised by the Healthcare Commission, which then feed into Trusts' rankings
- Local Involvement Networks (LINks), which have been introduced to enable communities to influence healthcare services at a local level (these used to be called "Patient forums")
- The Foundation Trust Board of Governors, elected by members of the local community. It has a say on who runs a hospital and how it should be run, including the services it can provide.

Using Information & IT

This aspect of clinical governance ensures that:

- Patient data is accurate and up to date
- Confidentiality of patient data is respected
- Data is increasingly used to measure the quality of outcomes (e.g. through audits) and to develop services tailored to local needs.

Staffing & Staff Management

This relates to the need for

- appropriate recruitment and management of staff,
- ensuring that underperformance is identified and addressed,
- encouraging staff retention by motivating and developing staff and
- providing good working conditions.

From the above explanations, you may have noted that some of the pillars are more directly related to the day-to-day responsibilities of a junior doctor:

- Clinical Effectiveness
- Audit
- Risk Management
- Education & Training

Whenever you discuss clinical governance in an answer, you may prefer to discuss these in more depth and simply mention the other three. You can remember these 4 key pillars with the mnemonic CARE.

Mnemonics

If you are the type of person who likes to remember information through the use of mnemonics, here are a couple which will enable you to remember all the components of clinical governance:

Patient & Public Involvement	Staff management
Information & IT	Patient & Public Involvement
Risk Management	Audit & IT
Audit	Risk Management
Training / Education	Effectiveness (Clinical)
Effectiveness (Clinical)	Information & IT
Staff management	Training / Education

Answering the question

When asked to talk generically about clinical governance, a good structure for your answer would be as follows:

- Brief definition of clinical governance in your own words
- State and define the four CARE pillars
- List the other three pillars (with brief explanations if you have time)
- Give brief examples where you have practised clinical governance

Alternatively, you could bring examples within each of the four CARE pillars instead of bringing them in at the end of the answer. Whatever you do, do not attempt to describe each of the pillars in detail. Discussing an introduction to clinical governance and 7 pillars in two minutes would allocate only 15 seconds per section. Not only are you unlikely to remember everything in the right order, but you will also find yourself speeding through your answer. It is better to talk knowledgeably and confidently about 4 pillars than to waffle about all 7.

9.25 What is your experience of clinical governance?

Be careful with questions on clinical governance because it is easy to regurgitate its definition and the 7 pillars without really answering the question. This question does not ask for a description of clinical governance, but for your own experience of it. The examiners will judge you on your overall understanding of governance, and the relevance and clarity of your examples. In order to achieve this, you must choose the pillars which are the most relevant for you, i.e. those which you are most likely to have had experience of. These would typically be the CARE pillars (see previous question).

Here are some questions which will help you think about your experience in each area of clinical governance:

Clinical Effectiveness

Have you:
- Played a role in implementing new guidelines or protocols in your department?
- Played a role in facilitating the use of guidelines in your department, for example by creating proformas or checklists?
- Initiated a change to an established protocol because you felt that it was inappropriate?
- Collated a set of guidelines (whether in hard copy or online)?
- Needed to do a literature search or read up on guidelines to determine the best care for a patient?
- Got any research experience?
- Published case reports or papers?

Audit

Have you:
- Participated in an audit?
- Had opportunities to improve clinical practice with one of your audits?
- Supervised others doing audits?
- Completed an audit, including making changes and re-auditing?

Risk Management

Do you:
- Double-check that you are doing the right thing (labels, dosages, etc.)?
- Seek help or advice from others appropriately?
- Encourage your juniors to come to see you if they have problems or if they have made mistakes?

- Show support towards juniors (rather than blame them) when they get things wrong? When this happens, do you consider how the system can be improved to ensure that mistakes do not happen again?
- Know what Root Cause Analysis is? This is a thorough investigation into the background surrounding a serious untoward event (critical incident), examining protocols, actions, personnel. One technique is the Five Whys: Why did that happen? And why did that happen? Etc.

Have you:
- Identified a problem with some aspects of care in your team and raised the issue with seniors (i.e. a protocol out of date, a common practice which is not wholly appropriate)?
- Reported any significant issues or near misses?
- Made a mistake or had a near miss that you then reported and discussed with colleagues (or maybe formally recorded through a critical incident form)?
- Dealt with a patient's complaint and ensured that practice changed as a result?

Education & Training

Do you:
- Have a personal development plan?
- Attend courses on a regular basis?
- Identify your weak areas and find ways of improving your skills?
- Read about cases you have seen, when you get back from work?
- Observe senior colleagues to learn from their practice?
- Ensure that you teach and train junior colleagues when the opportunity arises (and take the initiative to do so without being asked)?
- Read journals regularly?

Patient / Public involvement

Have you:
- Done an audit of patient satisfaction?
- Designed a questionnaire to obtain patient feedback?
- Sought informal feedback from patients on your/your department's performance?
- Been involved in responding to patient concerns about your service?
- Involved patients in the design of either a service or some teaching?

Using Information & IT

Do you:
- Anonymise data when you use it for audit or other purposes?
- Correct patient records when they are found to be inaccurate?

Have you:
- Queried data to identify trends and subsequently suggested changes to practice (maybe as part of an audit project)?
- Gained IT skills relating to data handling (e.g. databases, web)?

Staffing & Staff Management

Have you:
- Had to discuss performance issues with a colleague or had to report under-performance to senior colleagues?
- Taken steps to improve working relationships within a team in which you worked?
- Developed ways of improving relationships with other teams (e,g. nurses, other departments)?
- Made efforts to involve others in projects, when you felt they would benefit from such an involvement?

Delivering your answer

Once you have identified the extent of your experience, all you need to do is list each of your experiences using the pillars as your structure. For each experience, explain how this contributed towards governance and helped maintain or improve standards of care.

9.26 In your Trust, who is responsible for clinical governance?

This question is becoming more and more common, and usually comes as a probing question to a more substantial question on governance.

There are two levels of responsibility that you need to discuss:

- The legal responsibility
- The practical responsibility.

Legal responsibility

Since 1999, it is the Trust Board that is responsible for the quality of care provided by the Trust. That responsibility is exercised through the implementation of clinical governance. As head of the Trust Board, the Chief Executive of the Trust is ultimately the person who is accountable. Every year, each Trust must prepare an Annual Review of Clinical Governance. This summarises the quality of care and the implementation of good clinical governance.

Practical responsibility

Although the Chief Executive and the Trust Board are responsible, they obviously cannot do all the work by themselves. Their role is therefore to make sure that there are structures in place to ensure that clinical governance is fully embedded at all levels. The responsibility for clinical governance is delegated to the Medical Director, the Nursing Director, Clinical Directors, consultants and ultimately all staff. In fact, in an environment where infections such as MRSA and C.Difficile are causing so many problems, the cleaners play a role which is as important as anyone else's. Ultimately, everyone in the hospital is responsible for ensuring that standards of care are constantly maintained and improved.

Answering the question

When you answer the question, discuss the two levels of responsibility. Make sure that you include your own role in implementing clinical governance, using examples.

9.27 What is the difference between a standard, a guideline and a protocol?

This is another common question, which interviewers sometimes narrow down to the difference between a protocol and a guideline.

A standard is a defined level of quality that must be achieved. Standards are used to ensure that quality of care is maintained at the best possible level. Through the process of clinical audit, clinicians compare their own practice to the standards set by NICE, Royal Colleges or other associations and make appropriate adjustments to their practice to ensure that any underperformance that has been identified is remedied. Targets are also standards. For example, "by December 2004 all patients requiring emergency admission via the Emergency Department are admitted to a bed in the hospital, within four hours of arrival."

A guideline is a statement which is designed to assist clinicians in making decisions. Guidelines are recommendations for clinical practice based on evidence and the local infrastructure. They must be interpreted in the light of the particular patient and settings, as well as the strength of the evidence on which they are based.

A protocol is a step-by-step approach to dealing with an issue such as managing a patient, checking that the right patient/side is being operated on, dealing with a complaint, etc. Protocols must normally be followed exactly (unlike guidelines, which are subject to interpretation). Their purpose is to ensure that there is a systematic approach to dealing with important issues. For example, in Paediatric Oncology, almost all of the conditions have nationally-agreed protocols. These specify diagnostic criteria, investigations for diagnosis and monitoring (what and when), and treatment of the disease and any complications (again, what and when).

When you answer this question, give examples of each type based on your practice. As much as possible, choose examples from the specialty to which you are applying (if you don't, they will most likely ask you to quote some, so be prepared).

9.28 How do you critically analyse a paper?

What is critical analysis?

The purpose of evidence-based medicine is to determine how a patient should be managed based on best available evidence, the clinician's own clinical judgement and patient values (see 9.20). To determine what constitutes best evidence, it is essential to understand the papers which are published, the value they add to the pool of evidence, the flaws they present, their validity and their applicability to your patient. The critical appraisal process (i.e. the systematic analysis of a paper) is designed to enable clinicians to draw appropriate conclusions about the usefulness and validity of the published evidence.

How does critical analysis feature at interviews?

At the interview you may simply be asked how you would critically analyse a paper. You may also be asked to critically appraise a real paper. In such cases, you will be asked to come early in the day and will be given time to prepare. Typically, preparation time is 45 to 60 minutes and you will have 10 to 20 minutes to present your critical appraisal. Once you have presented your critical appraisal of the paper, the interviewers may ask questions on the paper itself and the issues it raises. You may also be asked questions on the different types of research and on statistics.

Everyone has their own technique to critically appraise papers, the easiest approach being to go through each section from top to bottom, addressing relevant points as you go. Whichever process you follow, your aim will be to address the key issues which are set out below:

General background

Title:
- Is the title relevant in relation to the content?

Journal:
- Is it peer-reviewed?

Impact factor of the journal:
The impact factor is a measure of how frequently articles in the journal are cited. A higher impact factor suggests that the journal is more learned and has higher quality content. One needs to remember, however, that it is also related to the specialty. Most specialist journals are likely to have lower impact factors than general medical journals, and subspecialty journals will have lower impact factors again.

Authors:

- Which institution are they from? Is it a noteworthy academic institution?
- How many authors are there, e.g. is it a multicentre study with a lot of academic influence?
- Who are the authors? Are they renowned or credible in their field? Are there any non-academic or renowned statisticians in the list?
- Are the authors associated with drug companies?
- Has the research been sponsored by an institution with a vested interest?

Submission:

- How much time elapsed between original submission date and publication? In some papers the date of original submission is shown. A very long time between original submission and acceptance would suggest a lot of reworking.

Introduction

- Do the authors clearly lay out the background to the study as being worthy of investigation?
- Is the study particularly novel in comparison to what has already been published in the literature?
- Are the aims and hypothesis clearly set out?

Methods

Researchers may say this is the most important part of the paper since this is the basis of the scientific approach that was used. This will vary depending on whether it is a case-controlled (snap shot) or cohort study (following up people over a period of time).

- What is the overall study design: case study, case-controlled, cohort study? Is this an interventional study where a treatment or procedure is applied to one or more groups and results are measured subsequently?

  - If a review, was it systematic or a meta-analysis?
  - For a drug treatment: was it a randomised controlled trial?
  - For study of prognosis, was this a cohort study?
  - For study of causation, was this a case-controlled study?

- Was data collected prospectively or retrospectively? If retrospectively, it has greater chance for error if one is relying on data recorded prior to the conception of the study.

Although expert opinions exist in the literature, the main studies to be appraised would be those involving numerous subjects, i.e. case-controlled or cohort. In addition, the best form of evidence comes from meta-analyses where randomised controlled trials (cohort) are compared. However, this involves complex statistics or calculations to ensure that studies of often similar designs are presented in a comparable fashion. If you are required to comment on these, it would be more in terms of the suitability of the individual studies to be compared as a group and for you to interpret the final analysis, e.g. the combined odds or hazard ratios of an intervention or risk on final outcome.

Case-controlled studies

- Was this a single-centred or multicentre study?
- Were there few or multiple study investigators?
- Were the case definitions and outcome measures accurately and appropriately defined?
- Were the clinical measures appropriately reproducible by all study measurements?
- Were cases appropriately matched to the controls? You may wish to look at subject characteristics such as demographics and other biometric values – are they explicitly documented in the report?

Randomised controlled trials (RCTs)

These are likely to form the majority of articles that you would be asked to appraise. Usually they involve two or more study groups, followed up over time and differing only in the intervention (procedure or drug therapy they receive).

It is important that the study is well controlled and the groups differ only in the intervention. So:

- How were the subjects recruited? Was this random or consecutive?
- Are there any possibilities of bias in the recruitment process? Were measures added to specifically remove human choice and bias?
- What were the inclusion criteria? Did they include individuals who would innately bias the results of the intervention?
- What were the exclusion criteria? Did they exclude individuals for whom you would wish to know the impact of this intervention?
- Are the study groups large enough? The strength of any association will be measured statistically and this will depend on the size of the studies sampled. Often a "power" calculation is made before the study is undertaken, which guides the researchers in determining the optimum size of the study groups needed to reach a desired strength of significance.
- Was each of the study groups treated in the same way, with the exception of the intervention? This may include follow-up visits, number of measurements/investigations/scans, centre in which they receive their care, personnel they were in contact with, etc.
- Are the groups well matched for baseline characteristics? Often a table is shown detailing demographics and other biometric values – are there any characteristics missing from this table that you feel relevant, e.g. smoking, BMI, etc.
- Was length of follow-up adequate? Some outcome measures are rare and a long follow-up is required to await their manifestation.

- What were the study's end points (outcome measures): were they appropriate for the question being asked? For example, coronary events measured by clinical symptoms or ECG or cardiac enzymes – was this the same for both groups? This may not be the case in a multicentre study.
- What was the dropout rate? Was this unacceptably high thereby reducing the statistical power of those remaining in the study groups?
- How are dropouts and missing values accounted for statistically, i.e. was this an "on-treatment analysis" where only the results of those still on treatment at the end are evaluated or is this an "intention to treat" analysis where every subject's results are noted whether they continued with the intervention or not? In this case the researchers have to decide what they do with subjects who changed intervention (switched drugs) or dropped out or died. This has to be clearly stated. A common example is "missed drug = failure". So the number of dropouts will be relevant when studying the overall supposed effect in that study arm.

Results

- Are the results for all of the end points stated clearly (tabulated or graphically represented)?
- What statistical methods were used? Were they appropriate for the type of data collected, i.e. for continuous or discrete data – parametric or non-parametric methods?
- For data points in text, tables or graphs, were adequate confidence intervals calculated, i.e. to the 95% level? How wide are these confidence intervals? Is there overlap with the comparator groups?
- What is the p-value? This is the chance (between 0 and 1) that the observed event occurred by chance. By convention, a p-value less than 0.05 (i.e. a 1 in 20 chance) is deemed significant.

Conclusions

The conclusion section should only discuss the findings stated in the results section. The authors must not present any new data in the conclusion section.

- The conclusions should be discussed in terms of association of the intervention or risk factor with the outcome measure. This association is only confirmed if the odds ratios of p-values are significantly strong, i.e. the usual cut-off for a p-value is less than 0.05 with the smallest p-values giving the greatest strength of association. Authors sometimes discuss "trends" where there is an apparent association in the data, yet the p-value is close to but not smaller than 0.05. It is acceptable for authors to state this but one should be wary if most of their conclusions hang on trends of relatively large p-values.
- Some reviewers negatively critique papers in which many factors are analysed for association. These may be colloquially termed "fishing exercises", the criticism being (i) some of the positive findings were not the primary objec-

tives of the study and (ii) the more variables that are analysed from a data set, the greater the likelihood that an association may be found purely by chance.

- Where associations are strong the authors will suggest a possible causation between intervention or risk factor and outcome measure. Are these causations scientifically plausible? Are they justified by putative mechanism of action or appropriate time relationship between cause and effect? Does this agree with findings of other research in this field?
- Do the authors make claims which you feel are appropriate or inappropriate regarding the evidence they have presented?
- Do they translate these findings to be applied to situations/populations which you feel are reasonable or unreasonable?
- Are study limitations discussed? Are suggestions for future study refinement or extension work mentioned?
- Have appropriate plans been made for future study?

And finally

- Have the authors accepted or rejected their hypothesis, i.e. has this paper proven something to you? And crucially:
- Does any of this apply to the populations or individuals you care for?
- Will this change your management in any way?

9.29 Systematic review, meta-analysis & randomised controlled trials (RCTs)

Whilst discussing a paper you may be asked probing questions about the different possible designs for research studies, such as "What is a randomised controlled trial?" or "What is a meta-analysis?". In this chapter, we set out the different types of designs and their key features.

Systematic review & meta-analysis (Evidence Level Ia)

A systematic review is a review and summary of the existing high-quality research evidence relating to a given topic. Systematic reviews constitute the highest level of evidence for evidence-based medicine purposes. There is a standardised method for conducting systematic reviews. Researchers will seek to include all relevant material, including non-English work, unpublished papers and research from different databases. They will contact lead researchers and ask if they know of other publications that should be included.

Relevant studies are often combined using meta-analysis. The best known collection of systematic reviews is the Cochrane Collaboration.

A meta-analysis is a way of combining the results from several related studies into some form of standardised measure of effect size. By combining and adjusting the results from a collection of studies, giving appropriate weighting to the various studies involved, a meta-analysis will produce stronger evidence. On the negative side, the end result will only be as good as the material used for the meta-analysis: good meta-analysis of flawed research studies would result in flawed results.

Randomised controlled trial (Evidence Level Ib)

Randomised controlled trials (RCTs) are studies in which the interventions are randomly allocated to patients in order to ensure that known and unknown confounding factors are evenly distributed between treatment groups. The word "controlled" refers to the fact that patients are not studied in isolation, but by reference to a "control group". The control group is given the old (or standard) treatment, a placebo that looks similar to the new treatment or no treatment at all.

Different types of control groups

- No-treatment concurrent control groups – subjects are randomly allocated the test treatment or no treatment.

- Placebo concurrent control group – subjects are randomly allocated the test treatment or a similar-looking treatment which does not contain the active element.

- Active control group – subjects are randomly allocated the test treatment or another form of treatment. This type of control group tends to be used to demonstrate the superiority of one treatment over another.

- Dose response control group – subjects are randomly allocated to different doses of the test treatment (this may include a zero dose, i.e. a placebo).

- External control and historical control – the test group is being compared to a group of patients who are external to the study. This may be a group of patients from an earlier study or a group of patients treated contemporaneously but in a different setting.

- Crossover trials – the two treatments are switched between the two groups (after a washout period) to see which one has a better effect on any particular patient, i.e. the patient is the control.

Open vs. blind trials

- Open trials are trials where both the researcher and the patient knows which treatment the patient has been allocated. It is difficult to remove bias since the patient knows whether he is being given a placebo or not. There are, however, situations where the patient needs to know what treatment is being administered as does the doctor (for example, in the case of surgical procedures).

- Single-blind trials are trials where the researcher knows which treatment is being given to which patient, but where the patient does not know. The main drawback of this approach is that the researcher may subconsciously affect the outcome for the patient, treating and informing patients slightly differently in view of his knowledge.

- Double-blind trials are trials where neither the researcher, nor the patient, knows which treatment the patient has been allocated. Whenever there are viable alternatives, double-blind trials are the preferred option because they remove any bias. When the person administering the treatment is also unaware of which group the patient is in, this may be termed "triple-blind".

10 Difficult colleagues

What are the interviewers testing?

The interviewers will use these questions to test a range of skills and behaviours, including:

- Being safe: patients should be your first priority and the interviewers will want to know that you are not placing yourself or your colleagues before patient safety.

- Your understanding of the dilemmas that the situation presents. These questions are difficult because there isn't always a single answer. For example, there are rumours about a colleague taking drugs in his spare time. You could argue that it is none of your business, but it may develop into something more serious and place patients at risk. You will need to demonstrate that you understand the different perspectives and that you are able to decide on an appropriate course of action.

- Your approach to the problem: many candidates think that telling the clinical director will resolve the problem. There are often times, however, when the problem can be resolved without going to senior colleagues (e.g. if the subject has only been late a couple of times). In any case, seniors will generally prefer you to "bring solutions, rather than problems". There are times where it is necessary to involve a senior colleague and this should be handled sensitively. The interviewers will be looking at the thought processes that you demonstrate.

- Your communication skills and empathy: some scenarios may contain a more human element, i.e. where the behaviour exhibited by the colleague is potentially linked to a personal problem. In other scenarios, the situation could be very delicate and seriously backfire if communication is not handled properly. The interviewers will be keen to know that you can handle these matters sensibly and communicate appropriately.

- Your team approach: it is unlikely that you will be able to sort out the problem by yourself. The interviewers will therefore want to determine to what extent you involve other people from the team, and how appropriate that involvement is.

Answering the question

Questions on problem colleagues may look different on the surface but once you have learnt to answer a few of them you will know how to approach pretty much any scenario thrown at you. In order to make best use of the material contained in this chapter, it is important that you familiarise yourself with the SPIES structure (see 5.3). It will form the backbone of your answer. In order to provide an effective answer, you willl also need to follows the following principles:

Avoid providing answers that are too robotic and algorithmic
Although ready-made structures are extremely useful to ensure that you don't forget any salient points, it is also crucial that you use your common sense whenever you answer any question relating to practical situations. You do not handle a drunken consultant in the same way that you would handle a junior colleague who is often late. Keep things in perspective and use your common sense.

Explain the "how" and the "why", not just the "what"
Most candidates "know" the answers to all these "difficult colleague" questions. However, not many deliver answers which are interesting to listen to. After 15 candidates, the interviewers will be bored of hearing the same thing time after time. In order to provide an answer which is different and highlights your maturity, you will need to mention all the essential steps and why you would act that way.

For example, you may feel that the situation needs to be escalated to the clinical director. Why is that and how would you handle that process?

- Will you discuss the matter with the problem doctor first or not? If not, why not? And if yes, what will you be achieving by doing this?

- Is the clinical director the best person to contact? What about the colleague's educational supervisor or another consultant? Which is better and why?

- Will you actually be formally discussing the matter with a senior colleague or will you simply raise it informally with them? Why? What are you seeking to achieve?

- You will no doubt need to demonstrate that you can support the colleague in question as well as your team in dealing with the problem. How will you do that and why?

My experience is that candidates take an approach that is far too theoretical when they answer questions on difficult colleagues. To ensure that your answer is natural, try to imagine what you would do if this were a real situation. In other words, stop thinking of the question as an "interview" question and start picturing yourself in a real-life scenario. Use your common sense.

If possible, highlight the dilemmas at the start of your answer

Once you have been given a scenario, you should be able to determine very quickly what problems the situation poses. If possible, you should present these at the very start of the answer so that your interviewers know how you are approaching the problem.

For example, if you have to deal with the "drunk consultant" question, you could start your answer with a statement such as "There are two problems that this scenario poses. I will need to make sure that patients are safe but I also need to make sure that the problem is handled sensitively so that the consultant does not suffer any more embarrassment than he has already caused."

This will give an idea of the direction that you are taking and will also reassure the interviewers that you are thinking rationally about the problem rather than just regurgitating some standard answer.

Avoid providing specific examples in the main body of the answer

Some of you may have had experience of dealing with problems similar to the scenario that the question is addressing. If this is the case, do not mention them before you have dealt with the generality of the question. If you go straight into a specific example, you will spend all your time on it and will miss out some vital parts of the answer, which may not have featured prominently in the real-life situation that you dealt with.

10.1 One of your consultants comes on the ward drunk one morning. What do you do?

What you are trying to achieve?

Your main objectives in dealing with this situation will be to ensure that:

- patient safety is assured
- the consultant is safe
- seniors are aware so that action can be taken to prevent the problem from recurring and to ensure that the issues which led the consultant to become drunk are being addressed
- the consultant is supported in dealing with these issues
- the whole situation is handled sensitively.

Applying the SPIES structure (see 5.3)

Seek information
There is little information you need to gather if you are actually present when the consultant comes in. The question is telling you that he is drunk so there is no information you can gather which would make a difference to the way in which you handle the matter. The outcome of the investigation may, however, be altered if he has been affected temporarily by a divorce or bereavement.

Patient safety.
If the consultant is drunk then he is a danger to patients and should be taken away from the clinical environment. In this case the clinical area is the ward, but the question could equally refer to a theatre.

There are many ways in which you could remove the consultant from the clinical area but, however you do it, you must make sure that you do it in the quickest and most sensitive manner so as to minimise the impact on patients and the embarrassment to the consultant and to the team.

You may want to try the following approaches (in decreasing order of suitability):
- Talk to the consultant and convince him to leave and go home
- Involve another senior member of the team (another consultant or even a senior nurse) who may have more influence than you on the consultant. Remember that you are trying to handle the matter sensitively, therefore you would need to involve someone that the consultant trusts in order to minimise conflict.
- A senior member of an adjacent team. Typically this would be another consultant.
- Security (as a very last resort – hopefully you will have found someone to help you before you reach this stage).

Once the consultant has left the clinical area, you will need to make sure that any actions or decisions made by that consultant are reviewed and that any patients he has seen are followed up appropriately.

Initiative

Is there any action that you could undertake by yourself (i.e. before you involve anyone else) to resolve or help the situation at your level? In the case of a drunken consultant, it would be inappropriate for you to attempt to resolve the entire problem by yourself; however, there are a number of useful steps that you can take such as:

- Making sure that the consultant is safe, i.e. that he goes home safely by taxi or sleeps it off in the doctors' mess. Make sure that he doesn't drive home and check that he has arrived safely.

- Informing the person in charge that the consultant was unwell and needed to go home so that appropriate cover can be arranged.

- Volunteering to cover some of consultant's duties, which might otherwise be neglected. At a junior level, you might not be able to take on the responsibilities that the consultant would have handled, but you can work with the team to share the workload and ensure that patient care is being appropriately provided.

Escalate

If the consultant turns up drunk, then there is no doubt that this shows a lack of insight – despite being drunk, he failed to realise that he could constitute a danger to patients. His judgement is questionable and he therefore poses a risk to patients, not only in the present, but also in future if he has or develops an alcohol addiction.

As a result, you would be expected to raise the matter with an appropriate senior colleague. You would want to avoid contacting too many people so as not to spread rumours and undermine the reputation of the problem consultant. You really need to contact someone who is likely to have some influence over the situation; this would typically be the clinical director or a senior consultant who can take the problem on board and start dealing with it.

From then on, you have effectively transferred the responsibility of dealing with the problem to senior colleagues. However, although this probably means that your input will no longer be required to deal with the core of the matter, you still have a responsibility to raise the alarm if you feel that the senior response is inadequate.

Support

The consultant's behaviour is likely to have its roots in some kind of personal problem. In addition, the incident is likely to have consequences, if not for his career, at least on his credibility. You should therefore show as much support as you can towards him (more so if you know him well). You should also ensure that you support your team in dealing with consequences of the problem; for example you may need to take on extra duties temporarily until the consultant gets better.

Follow-up questions

Interviewers often ask follow-up questions to test your understanding of your responsibilities and duties as a doctor. Follow-up questions typically include:

- "Once you have reported the problem to the clinical director, what is likely to happen?" (see 10.2)
- "What would you do if the drunken consultant asks you not to mention anything to anyone, because it was the first time that it happened and he promises it won't happen again?" (see 10.3)
- "If, after reporting the matter to the clinical director, you find that he is not responding appropriately, what would you do?" (see 10.4).

10.2 Once you have reported the problem to the clinical director, what is likely to happen?

This is a question which can be asked in many ways, either generally (i.e. according to the wording above) or more specifically (such as "Which external bodies is the clinical director likely to involve in order to resolve the situation?").

You can also structure the answer to this question according to the SPIES structure:

Seek information
The clinical director will want to gather information about the incident from you, from other colleagues who may have been present at the time and also from the consultant who was drunk. He will also want to learn, from others, whether similar incidents have occurred in the past.

Patient safety
The clinical director will need to make a decision as to the extent to which patient safety is endangered by the consultant and will need to take appropriate steps. This may include removing the consultant from certain duties or suspending him during the investigation. This is a decision that will need to be taken at Trust level following discussion with the medical director.

Initiative
The clinical director will need to ensure that patient care is covered adequately whilst the problem is being resolved. He will need to discuss with other colleagues how the team should be reorganised to deal with the consultant's enforced absence.

The clinical director will also seek to understand the reasons behind the consultant's behaviour. In particular, he should establish whether the problem is linked to some form of personal problem, stress at work or any other problem for which the consultant can be supported.

Escalate
In view of the seriousness of the incident, its potential impact on patient safety and on the reputation of the Trust, the clinical director will most likely engage in a discussion with the medical director (i.e. his direct superior, who represents the clinical side on the Trust's Board). They will together, perhaps in consultation with the chief executive, decide how they should proceed. They may decide that the incident can be closed with a simple (but final) warning or they may move for suspension and reporting to the GMC.

Support
The level of support provided by seniors to the consultant will depend on the nature of the problem:

- If the drinking has nothing to do with an ongoing alcohol abuse problem, senior colleagues may be less understanding than if there is a real personal problem.

- If the drinking has a personal cause (e.g. personal problems, stress at work) the clinical director may wish to offer support to the colleague to help him cope. This may include simply giving him additional time off or even restructuring the way he works.

- If the drinking is a habit, then the clinical director should encourage the colleague to seek help from appropriate support groups. In some cases, this may even be a condition of the consultant's return to work.

10.3 What would you do if the drunken consultant asks you not to mention anything to anyone because it was the first time that it happened and he promises he won't happen again?

Your duty

The fact that he has turned up drunk raises concern about patient safety. Even if the consultant has not touched a single patient that day, the fact that he lacked insight about his own fitness to practise is worrying by itself. He should have recognised that he was unfit, called in sick and stayed at home. You therefore have no choice. You <u>must</u> report the matter to a senior colleague.

Communicating with the consultant

You are facing someone who is obviously trying hard to limit the damage that he has caused to himself and you must be empathetic towards his situation. Whilst you should be firm in asserting that you have no choice, you should also try to be supportive and convey the message that, ultimately, if he has some form of problem, it will be best resolved with everything in the open. The best you can offer is your support and understanding.

Think of the worst-case scenario

Some candidates argue that "it is harsh to report someone, if it is the first time they have made a mistake". If you think this, consider what would happen if the consultant comes in drunk again, but this time harms or even kills a patient. An investigation would be launched and it would quickly be established that it had happened before, but you kept quiet. This would get you into serious trouble. Therefore you cannot take the risk and you should report it to a senior colleague.

10.4 If, after reporting the matter to the clinical director, you find that he is not responding appropriately, what would you do?

A simple answer

If the clinical director is failing to act, then he may be unfit to practise because he is letting other doctors potentially harm patients. Therefore, in accordance with the GMC's *Good Medical Practice*, you will need to report the matter to an appropriate senior colleague: in this case, the medical director. If the medical director fails, you will need to go to the chief executive and after that to the GMC. This is the answer that most interviewers would be looking for and which, in most circumstances, would give you the maximum mark for this question.

However, although this would be an absolutely correct answer to give, some candidates have received feedback that the interviewers were looking for a "more refreshing answer". To provide a more comprehensive answer you can use the SPIES structure.

A more comprehensive answer

Seek information
Accusations must be based on objective information. For example, you may have observed further patterns of unsafe behaviour. Make a note and enquire with other colleagues if need be (discreetly).

Patient safety
If there are further unsafe episodes, then you must ensure that patient safety is preserved. This may involve confronting the consultant about the recurrent problem. You may also have to discuss the problem with other senior colleagues.

Initiative
The fact that you believe that the clinical director is not responding appropriately does not actually mean that he has been completely ignoring the problem. He may have tried to resolve the problem, but struggled to deal with that consultant and is currently working on alternative plans. You should not jump to conclusions. If you remain concerned about the perceived lack of progress, it would be appropriate to return to the clinical director and ask what has happened. The clinical director might then explain to you how he is handling the situation. If you feel that your concerns are not being taken seriously, then you should escalate.

Escalate
If you feel that you are being ignored or that the action taken is insufficient, then you need to take your concerns to the medical director and, if necessary, to the chief executive.

Whatever you do, never escalate without having first exhausted discussions at each level. For example, if you have a problem with the clinical director, raise it with him first before going to the medical director. Also never raise your concerns with people like the media as you would undermine the authority of your superiors (those who genuinely care) and you may also undermine patient confidence in their local Trust. This would be counterproductive and you may in fact make things worse overall.

If you do not know how to handle the issue, then you can seek advice from your defence union (Medical Defence Union or Medical Protection Society), NCAS or even the GMC.

Support
Ultimately, patient care is what matters most; so you should continue to support your team in dealing with patients, despite all the problems that are taking place. You should also continue to support the problem doctor.

10.5 One of your junior colleagues has been late for 20 minutes every day for the past 4 days. What do you do?

This is another question about a problem colleague, and therefore we suggest using the SPIES structure.

Seek information
There may be different reasons why the colleague is late. Maybe he has discussed this with a senior colleague previously but simply failed to inform you about it. Maybe he is having personal problems which he does not wish to share with others. Maybe his train is late due to engineering works. Maybe he is new to the hospital and is travelling long distances. Or maybe he has an attitude problem.

With a lot of "maybes", you really need to seek some information about the nature of the problem. This can be done by approaching the colleague and gently asking whether there is anything you can help with. You can add that you have noticed he has had trouble getting to work on time.

Patient safety
A delay of 20 minutes is unlikely to cause major concern towards patient safety. In most cases, it will have an impact on the team without necessarily impacting on safety. However, there may be cause for concern if:

- the colleague is missing handovers and provides substandard care
- the colleague is carrying the crash bleep and is not always available
- the colleague rushes jobs to make up for his lateness.

If this is the case, then you should raise these concerns with a clinic or ward manager or any senior colleague so that they can take action. You should also ensure that patient safety is not affected. This may mean ensuring that you take on some of his jobs or place at handovers.

Initiative
It is possible that the problem is due to a temporary problem such as family problems or train delays. If the problem is likely to be very short term and you are reassured that your colleague has tried his best to sort things out, then you may wish to show a little flexibility by covering for him for the period of the delay and also by recommending that he should discuss his problems with a senior colleague or a manager so that they can arrange a more flexible working pattern temporarily. Whatever you agree with your colleague should be shared with someone more senior. The manager may suggest a contract which makes expectations transparent for both parties.

Escalate

If you feel that the problem is affecting patient safety, that there is a lack of insight or that it is likely to persist, you will need to involve a consultant more formally.

Support

If the issue is linked to a family problem, then your colleague will appreciate your personal support during this difficult period.

The answer to this question requires more consideration than for the underperforming colleague. Due to the strong likelihood that the delay is linked to personal issues, your answer should reflect this by placing an equal emphasis on flexibility and support, and on raising the matter with senior colleagues.

10.6 Whilst in the mess, you see a bag of what looks like cocaine drop from your Registrar's pocket. What do you do?

This question works along a similar line to the others (i.e. you can answer it using the SPIES structure (see 5.3) except that, this time, you only have a suspicion rather than actual proof).

Dealing with the lack of certainty

When you deal with a drunken colleague, the impact on patient safety is clear and, once you have ensured that patients are safe, you need to report your concerns. However, in the case of a bag of cocaine falling out of your Registrar's pocket, there are some unknowns; for example:

- Is it actually cocaine? You could of course enquire with your colleague but he is unlikely to own up to it.
- Assuming it is cocaine, is your colleague actually taking any? He could be carrying it for someone else. He might even be selling it on.

You don't know whether this matter is impacting on patient care and your colleague's safety as a doctor. For this reason, you cannot take the risk of letting the matter go and, on the basis that you are not the best person to investigate this issue, you will need to report it to senior colleagues. If, after investigation, the matter is nothing to worry about (maybe it was just sugar!) then everyone will just move on. However, if the matter is serious then the seniors will be able to handle it properly because you have brought it to their attention.

"Raising the matter with seniors seems harsh"

Some may argue that reporting the matter with seniors is harsh. It may be the case (particularly if it was not cocaine after all), but you need to weigh this against the alternatives. Sorting this out directly with the colleague will most likely lead you nowhere (since he will undoubtedly deny it) and, in any case, it would only lead to a temporary solution (you can't keep an eye on the colleague every single day – it is not your job). Doing nothing would actually be unsafe. Not only might he be under the effects of cocaine at work, but also the drug abuse may be linked to stress or personal problems. These may be affecting your colleague's performance. Your success in handling the matter well will rest in the sensitivity that you demonstrate through your communication with everyone involved.

10.7	You wrote a case report for publication, which you gave to one of your consultants for review. After 2 weeks, he gives it back to you with two additional names as authors: his brother's and his wife's. What do you do?

Issues raised by the question

The issues in this question are as follows:

- The consultant lacks integrity by adding the names of two people (his brother and wife) who not only have not contributed to the case (if they did contribute to the case then there is absolutely no problem), but are two other doctors out there who have a CV with potentially fake information and may be getting jobs under false pretences. The fact that it is only a case report may not seem a big deal, but this indicates a certain frame of mind and they may well be faking other aspects of their CV. This does not reflect well on the consultant's integrity as a doctor.

- Having more authors undermines your own efforts as it dilutes your involvement.

On both counts, patient safety is not immediately affected, i.e. there is no reason to act that very minute, but it does raise some important questions. The best way to deal with it is as follows (following the SPIES structure):

Seek information
Discuss with the consultant why he has added the two names. Raise your concerns and try to get a sensible explanation from him.

Patient safety
No immediate action required. Patient safety is not immediately affected.

Initiative
Try to convince the consultant that this is wrong. Try to get him to change his mind. If you can, you should stand your ground and insist that the names are taken off. If the consultant has already given you the corrections back then you may take the initiative to send the case report off to the journal without the two names in question.

Escalate
If the situation is not easily resolved then you may consider raising the issue with another consultant or the clinical director.

Support
Not relevant here.

Follow-up question

Whenever candidates have been asked this question, it was followed up by the following question: "The consultant is your MMC referee and may give you a bad reference if you contest. How do you handle the situation?"

In answer to this question, if you are really worried about your reference then you need to discuss the matter with someone else at a senior level. They should arrange for another referee to take over. If there is no time to arrange another referee they should discuss the reference with the consultant in question beforehand to make sure that you do not suffer from the consequences.

10.8	Your consultant is managing a patient against the recommendations of the established guidelines. What do you do?

This question looks like a question on a difficult consultant but combines it with your knowledge of evidence-based practice and more specifically your understanding of the definition of a "guideline" (see 9.27)

Seek information
Before you jump to conclusions, you need to understand why the consultant is making the decision to go against the guideline. After all, he has several more years' experience and his decision is most likely to be correct.

The process of evidence-based medicine combines many more aspects than just the guideline. In particular the consultant's clinical judgement and the patient's values have to be taken into account. Consequently there are many reasons why the consultant may have taken his decision. For example:

- The guideline may not be suitable for the patient
- The consultant may be aware of recent evidence which would supersede the guideline (though the guideline has not yet been changed to allow for that evidence)
- The guideline may be suitable but the patient may have refused the recommended treatment.

Whatever the situation, the consultant should be in a position to educate you about his decision. The easiest way to approach him without sounding confrontational is to raise with him the fact that you are struggling to understand the decision that is being made and would like to discuss it with the consultant from an educational perspective.

Hopefully, by that time, you will be reassured that he is making the right decision.

Ensure patient safety at all costs. Escalate if necessary
If, after obtaining further information from the consultant, you feel uncomfortable about the proposed management then you must raise your concerns: in the first instance with the consultant, and, if needed, with another consultant. If you cannot get hold of another consultant, talk to the clinical director or another colleague.

Don't forget that you could also be wrong. So, if you have doubts, you always have the opportunity to discuss the issue with colleagues at your level or look things up. Also, remember not to contradict the consultant in front of patients. Any disagreement should be raised away from patients.

If the situation is an emergency and you do not have time to ask for a second opinion or engage in a discussion, then you will have no choice but to let the consultant go with his decision but you <u>must</u> record your disagreement in writing in the patient notes. This way, if there is a problem, you will not be blamed for not trying to resolve the initial problem.

Learn from the situation
If the consultant ended up being correct then you must ensure that you take steps to learn from that situation. You might want to read up on related matters or discuss the case at a teaching session.

10.9 Your consultant has made a mistake as a result of an error of judgement and is asking you to alter the patient's notes to match his version of events. What do you do?

There is no possible motive that could justify the consultant's behaviour. By not reporting the matter, you would not only help the consultant cover up for his mistake but you would also expose other patients to harm by not ensuring that action is taken against the consultant.

Seek information
There is no information to gather here as the nature of the problem is obvious.

Patient safety
Ensure that whatever mistake has been committed has been resolved and that the patient is safe (if the mistake did not result in death).

Initiative
Refuse to comply with the consultant's request and explain that it is unethical. You should also make a written record of the conversation that you are having with the consultant as your testimony may be required if any further action is taken.

Escalate
This issue is too serious for you to handle on your own. The consultant's behaviour is placing patients at risk and poses questions about his integrity. You should report the matter to the clinical director at the first opportunity. If he is not available or refuses to deal with the issue, escalate the matter to the medical director and thereafter to the chief executive.

Support
There is no support to give here, other than maybe towards the team in dealing with a situation where a consultant has gone (since he will most likely be suspended if your claims prove true).

10.10 During a ward round, your consultant shouts at you in front of a patient for getting an answer wrong. What do you do?

This is the type of question where it can be easy to get into automatic mode without thinking about the depth of the question, with an answer such as "This is bullying and therefore I will need to report it".

Yes, technically it is bullying and yes, it is unacceptable. However, your reaction will much depend on who the consultant is, whether he makes a habit of it, or whether it was just a normally pleasant consultant who became irritated on that day because of stress.

In your answer, you will therefore need to ensure that the unacceptability of the event is addressed, but also that you place the whole event into perspective and use your common sense.

Seek information
It is best not to allow the situation to escalate to full conflict, particularly in front of patients. In the first instance, you should simply shut up and arrange to meet the consultant after the ward round so that any discussion can be held in private. This will ensure that patients do not become witnesses to more conflict and also that an adult discussion can take place away from the emotions of the argument that took place in front of others. Once you are with the consultant, you must insist on an explanation for the shouting.

Patient safety
There is no patient "safety" issue as such here, but the patient's confidence in their medical care may have been undermined by the argument that they witnessed. You have also been embarrassed by the incident. In such circumstances, it would be appropriate for the consultant to talk to the patient themselves to apologise and reassure them. If the consultant does not want to do this, then you should take the initiative to do so yourself. If you feel uncomfortable about the whole idea or you feel that you may make things worse, you always have the option to talk to another consultant about it, who may be able to assist in the process.

Initiative
During the discussion with the consultant, if he has identified areas of concern about your performance, you should ask him how he feels you can resolve this. However, you should also remind him that it is never acceptable to put someone down in public, and even less so in front of patients. If you feel that you cannot do this, perhaps because the consultant is aggressive generally anyway, and that raising the matter directly with him would be counterproductive, then you still have the option of asking another consultant for advice (such as your educational supervisor, or any other consultant).

Escalate

If you feel threatened by the consultant or if this incident has become a bit of a habit, then you have to ensure that you discuss the problem with senior colleagues. In the first instance, the most obvious port of call would be your educational supervisor for advice, but you really ought to go straight to the clinical director as he is the person who is likely to have the most influence on the situation in terms of finding a lasting solution.

If this fails, then you should refer to the section in your employee manual/booklet dealing with bullying. That section will most likely tell you to report the matter in confidence either to the medical director or to someone from HR (each Trust is likely to have its own policy).

However, one thing is for sure: before you escalate the matter outside your team, you must take all possible steps to demonstrate that you have attempted to resolve the problem amicably within your team.

Support

This is not so relevant here. If anything, you are the one who needs to be supported. However, if the shouting was linked to stress or personal problems on the consultant's side then you should show some understanding (which is different to accepting the bullying!).

10.11 Your consultant does not seem interested in providing you with appropriate teaching. What do you do?

This question is perhaps more subtle than any other because it is nothing to do with clinical underperformance and immediate patient safety. Although the consultant is obviously not fulfilling his duties, the resolution of the problem will be a test of your communication skills and initiative more than your willingness to report the consultant quickly.

Seek information

There are two main reasons why the consultant may not be providing appropriate teaching. Either he just can't be bothered, or he is otherwise engaged and is finding it difficult to fit everything in.

Your first step will therefore be to determine the reasons why he is not providing any teaching. This is best addressed directly with the consultant in question. Because this is a teaching matter, you may first want to get together with other trainees to discuss the problem so that one of you approaches him with a mandate on behalf of the others. It may prove counterproductive to approach the consultant as a group because he may feel that you are ganging up on him.

Patient safety

Patient safety is not directly affected by the lack of teaching (in fact you probably spend more time with patients than you should) so there is no action needed on that front.

Initiative

Once you have organised a discussion with the consultant, you need to explain what you perceive the problem to be. This could be a simple lack of teaching time, a lack of protected time, or the fact that the teaching is there but lacks depth. During the discussion, you must acknowledge the constraints placed upon the department in relation to teaching (for example, lack of time due to European Working Time Directive) and avoid being over-critical. You must show a willingness to engage with the senior team to find a solution to the problem. Never forget that your aim is to find a solution to your problem, not to engage in confrontation for the sake of it.

In parallel to all this, you must show appropriate initiative to compensate for the lack of teaching by organising teaching with other consultants if you can, and by getting together with other trainees to organise study groups (if you are studying for exams, for example). It is of course important to get the problem consultant to provide teaching, but you cannot afford to wait until the problem is resolved to start training as you will waste your entire attachment.

So until the situation improves, make sure that you organise your own solutions too. In doing so, you will need to involve other Registrars or consultants anyway, which may provide a wake-up call to the team about the problem consultant.

Escalate

If, despite your best (and constructive) efforts, the situation is not evolving then you should broaden the discussion by involving your educational supervisor and perhaps other consultants. One idea may be to raise the matter of teaching in general at a team meeting (e.g. clinical governance meeting), avoiding mentioning the consultant in question but trying to get all seniors to agree on a training structure which is compatible with the level of service that needs to be provided to patients.

If the matter is stalling then you should also involve your clinical director, either directly or, preferably, through your educational supervisor (since he is responsible for your education and is also a consultant, which makes him an ideal person to deal with other consultants).

Support

There is no real support which needs to be brought to the consultant here, unless the lack of teaching is due to the fact that he is overstretched in other areas; in which case you may consider helping the team restructure its work so that the consultant's workload is alleviated.

In answering this question, the emphasis should be on discussion and negotiation. Make sure that you escalate to the appropriate people and do not escalate until you have tried every step to make the situation improve with the consultant first and then your educational supervisor.

10.12 You see one of your colleagues looking at child pornography on the mess's computer. What do you do?

This question can be dealt with successfully using the SPIES structure.

Seek information
Child pornography is not only illegal but your colleague also represents a possible danger to patients. Because of the seriousness of the situation, the issue will most certainly need to be discussed with a senior colleague. However, before you go down that route, you ought to discuss with the colleague in question what you saw. It may be a misunderstanding (i.e. perhaps it was simply a spam email that he received and opened, or perhaps a pop-up that he could not control) but it is difficult for you to investigate.

Patient safety
There is an obvious paediatric patient safety issue here, though it may not be immediate if the colleague is often working supervised or with other healthcare professionals. To ensure patient safety, for the immediate future, you should reassure yourself that the doctor is never on his own. You should also ensure that the matter is reported to a senior colleague as soon as possible so that further measures can be taken appropriately (e.g. suspension).

Initiative
So far, you have taken as much initiative as you could. Many candidates know that, for this question, the police need to be involved (since it is criminal) but this will really be a matter for the Trust to handle rather than you. By calling the police yourself, you may cause more harm than good in the short term (imagine the impact on your team and the patients if the police turned up on the ward to arrest the doctor!).

Escalate
Based on the above, your main responsibility will be to report the matter to a consultant or the clinical director as soon as possible. If the colleague is a consultant, then you should go to the clinical director. If the colleague is the clinical director then you should talk to the medical director. The seniors will deal with the matter, including ensuring that the police are being called.

Support
You may provide personal support to him through this ordeal and you should ensure that the matter is handled sensitively and confidentially.

10.13	A female patient, who saw one of your male colleagues last week, mentions in passing that the colleague in question examined their breast. This seems odd to you as there is no mention of such an examination in the notes and you see nothing which would justify a breast examination. What do you do?

This question was asked at Cardiology ST3 interviews but could be asked in more or less any specialty at any level using different types of unrecorded seemingly inappropriate behaviour.

The difficulty of the question lies in the uncertainty, i.e. whether your colleague simply forgot to document a genuine examination or whether he actually assaulted the patient. Once you have identified the nature of the problem, the course of action is fairly straightforward. To handle this question, use the SPIES structure:

Seek information
There are different possible reasons for this situation and you should avoid jumping to conclusions:

▪ Your colleague may have had a genuine concern about the patient's breast, perhaps based on a comment she made or something he observed. If this is the case then the examination may have been justified but it should have been recorded. There is nothing that indicates that the patient found it a problem but you may want to ask the patient whether she remember the circumstances behind the examination. This will give you an indication as to whether foul play was involved or not.

▪ Talking to the patient alone may not yield enough information, particularly if the patient ignores the reason behind the examination. You should try to talk to the colleague in question and also to anyone present in the room at the time. Hopefully, he would have had a chaperone. If he hasn't then this is another issue to address.

Essentially, you are trying to assess:
▪ Whether the breast examination was justified
▪ Whether the patient consented to it
▪ Why it was not recorded in the notes
▪ What the patient's feelings are about the situation. When talking to the patient, you should be careful not to express your concerns too openly as you may worry her unnecessarily. If anything needs to be communicated to the patient, this should be done once the situation has been clarified.

Patient safety
The safety of this particular patient is not immediately compromised since she is relating a past incident, though you may want to ensure that this particular patient is not seen by your colleague until further notice. You may also want to ensure that your colleague is appropriately chaperoned during examinations. See also the "Escalate" section.

Initiative
If the problem turns out to be a simple recording issue (i.e. the examination was genuine, the patient has consented but for whatever reason the examination was not recorded, perhaps because everyone was busy that day), then you may simply want to remind the colleague of the importance of recording as, in this particular incident, this could have had serious consequences.

If the examination was genuine but there was a problem in the communication with the patient, leading to the patient feeling confused after the event, then the issue is slightly more serious as the patient has effectively been examined intimately without consent. This may not be such a problem to resolve though, providing the patient is collaborating. The easiest thing to do may be to encourage your colleague to go to see a consultant with you so that you can all discuss the matter and find a solution. That solution might simply be to organise a meeting with the patient, your colleague and the consultant to explain the rationale behind the breast examination and to provide an apology, ensuring that the patient is okay about the whole incident. You should also encourage your colleague to contact his defence union in case the patient creates problems.

In addition, it may be constructive to use this incident to remind the team of the need for good notekeeping and the requirement to seek explicit consent, to be chaperoned and to check that the patient understands what is happening when consent is being sought. You could raise this in an email to the team, at a team meeting or a teaching session.

Escalate
If the problem turned out to be inappropriate behaviour by your colleague then you should report the matter to a consultant or the clinical director as soon as possible so that they can deal with the colleague. He would then most likely be suspended pending investigation.

Support
You should ensure that your colleague is supported throughout the situation.

Confidentiality, consent and other ethical principles

Occasionally, you may be asked questions relating to general ethics and its application to concrete scenarios. These questions could relate to issues as varied as difficult patients, complex consent issues or the management of an emergency with which you are unfamiliar.

The range of possible questions has no boundaries and your knowledge of ethics can be tested in different ways:

- By asking you factual questions about a key issue:
  - "What do you understand by the words 'Gillick competence'?"
  - "In which circumstances do you think it is acceptable to breach patient confidentiality?"

- By asking you how you would handle a specific situation, e.g:
  - a 14-year-old girl asking for a termination of pregnancy
  - an epileptic taxi driver who refuses to stop driving
  - an unconscious Jehovah's Witness who requires a blood transfusion.

- By engaging you in role play, with the patient being played by an interviewer or a trained actor.

Whatever the format, it is helpful to remember that all issues relate to four key principles. Therefore, rather than learn the management of individual situations by heart, concentrate on understanding and applying those key principles.

11.1 The four ethical principles of biomedical ethics

The following four principles are those used in biomedical science to guide decisions:

- **Beneficence**
  This word comes from the Latin "Bene" = Good and "Facere" = To do. Essentially it means that you must act in the patient's best interest.

- **Non-maleficence** (also, but rarely, called non-malfeasance)
  From the Latin "Male" = Bad and "Facere" = To do. You must not harm your patients. It is important to remember that many treatments may actually harm the patient (e.g. through side-effects) but what you need to keep in mind is the balance between benefit and harm.

- **Autonomy**
  From the Greek words "Auto" = Self and "Nomos" = Law, Custom.
  The patient has the right to choose what they want (i.e. whether to accept or refuse treatment).

- **Justice**
  Patients must be treated fairly. This principle deals mainly with the distribution of scarce resources and is particularly relevant when dealing with expensive drugs or procedures. It is the principle that may be applied to justify not giving a patient an expensive treatment if it means that a large number of patients then cannot benefit from other treatments as a result. However, in medicine, it is rarely used by doctors as decisions on drug availability are often taken at PCT/SHA level.

Whenever a dilemma occurs, it is because two or more of these principles clash. For example, a Jehovah's Witness refusing a blood transfusion will cause a clash between:

- Beneficence – transfusing is the best option to manage the patient
- Non-Maleficence – not transfusing may result in the patient's death
- Autonomy – the patient can choose what they feel is best for them.

Note: If the patient is competent, Autonomy always prevails over Beneficence and Non-Maleficence, i.e. the patient can do what they want with their body whether you think it will benefit them or harm them.

11.2	Confidentiality

The patient's right to confidentiality

The right to confidentiality is central to the doctor-patient relationship. It creates trust which makes patients feel safe to share information, without fear of that information being used inappropriately.

There are a number of simple measures that you can implement to ensure that patient confidentiality is protected (some of which may be discussed at interviews in specific patient-based scenarios). These include:

- Not leaving computers with patient records unattended
- Not leaving patient details showing on screen where they can be viewed by others
- Not letting patient notes lie around and not taking notes home with you unless they have been anonymised
- Not leaving handover sheets where they can be seen by patients and families
- Ensuring you check the identity of patients, particularly if you are discussing matters over the phone
- If the patient comes accompanied, asking the patient if they are comfortable with a third person sitting in on the consultation
- Not using the public as translators, even if they offer (e.g. unaccompanied, non-English speaker in the Emergency Department). There are a number of commercial interpreters available via telephone (e.g. LanguageLine)
- Carefully considering your reactions to questions asked by relatives or outside organisations (police, social services, etc.) when directed towards you.

Breaching patient confidentiality

Although patient confidentiality should be protected, there may be instances where it needs to be breached, some of which may be relevant to your daily practice.

The situations where breaching confidentiality is appropriate include:

- ***Sharing information with other healthcare professionals or others involved in the care of the patient***
  As a doctor, you constantly breach patient confidentiality by passing on information to other healthcare professionals. This may include sending a discharge summary to the patient's GP, or sending a referral letter to another doctor. It is accepted that such breaches are a routine aspect of patient management, providing the information is restricted to essential information. The patient is deemed to have provided implied consent. However, you must make sure that the patient understands that such disclosure of information is

being made and, if the patient objects to the disclosure, you must take every possible step to comply with their wishes.

- **Using information for the purpose of clinical audit**
  In order for the results of clinical audits to be meaningful, they include a representative sample of the patient cohort. It is therefore in the interest of good quality healthcare for patient data to be used for clinical audit. Providing patients have been informed that their data may be used internally for the purpose of audit and healthcare improvement, and providing they have not objected to its use, then you may use their data for the purpose of audit. This is a form of implied consent since you are not actually asking the patient to agree; you are simply informing them and allowing them to disagree, which rarely happens. If data is being given to external organisations for audit purposes, then the data must be anonymised. The data protection act also governs the way data is stored. Patients need to be informed which personal details are being held for audit or research purposes.

- **Disclosures required by law**
  There are a number of statutory requirements such as notifying a communicable disease, in accordance with the Public Health (Infectious Diseases) Regulations 1988. This includes measles, meningitis, mumps, tetanus and many others. The full list is available from the Health Protection Agency's website at www.hpa.org.uk. As always, you should make every effort to inform the patient, but their refusal cannot discharge you from your legal obligations.

- **Court order**
  You must disclose any information requested through a court order.

- **Disclosures to a statutory regulatory body**
  When investigating the fitness to practise of a health professional, regulatory bodies may require information about specific patient cases. Whenever possible you should discuss the disclosure of the information with the patients concerned. If discussing consent is not practical, or the patient refuses to give consent, then you need to discuss the situation with the regulatory body in question (e.g. GMC). They may judge that the disclosure is justified even without patient consent.

- **Disclosure in the public interest and to protect the patient or others from risk of serious harm or death**
  There may be cases where the benefit to society far outweighs the harm to the patient caused by the release of information:

  - In extreme cases of HIV patients knowingly infecting others
  - An epileptic driver who continues to drive, despite advice from the DVLA
  - Any case of very serious abuse where the victim is at serious risk of harm or death, even if they are a competent adult

- Notifying the presence of a sex offender
- A patient who is a doctor placing patients at risk through a medical condition (e.g. a surgeon with Hepatitis C).

- ***Treatment of children or incompetent adults***
This may happen when a child comes to see you, is not competent enough to make a decision, but is asking you to keep their visit confidential (the same would apply to any incompetent adult). In the first instance, you will need to negotiate with the patient to convince them to involve an appropriate person. If they refuse, then you may need to involve a third party anyway but only if you consider that the treatment is essential and in the patient's best interest. The patient should be aware of your intentions at all times.

- ***Abuse or neglect of an incompetent person***
The most common cases would be child or elderly abuse, or abuse of a patient with a mental illness.. If disclosure is in the best interest of the patient then you should do so promptly. If you decide not to report, you should be able to justify your decision. In fact, with child abuse, there is a duty to share information with other agencies, such as social care and the police. Therefore, if you suspect a child is about to make a disclosure, you should inform them that you will keep information confidential, unless they tell you something that you would need to share in order to protect their best interests.

Involving the patient

Whenever you need to breach confidentiality, you should always discuss it with the patient beforehand, obtain their consent and inform them of your plan. Although potentially a difficult conversation, it would certainly be easier than having to explain the breach afterwards. Being open and honest is generally appreciated by patients, even in challenging situations.

11.3 Competence and capacity

The difference between competence and capacity

Consent can only be taken from patients who are deemed to be "competent", i.e. who understand the information and are capable of making a rational decision by themselves. Competence is a legal judgement.

Doctors also frequently talk about "capacity to consent" or "mental capacity". This is a medical judgement. Capacity is formally assessed by doctors and nurses who must be sure that a patient is able to understand the proposed management, to comprehend the risks and benefits and to retain that information long enough to make balanced choices.

Because "competence" and "capacity" have similar meanings (in effect, a judge would rule as "competent" someone who has the capacity to make medical decisions), most doctors use them interchangeably.

Both competence and capacity are situation and time specific, i.e. they are determined at a particular point in time, in relation to a given treatment or procedure. So, for example, a patient may be competent enough to decide whether they agree to have their blood pressure taken, but not whether they should go ahead with a limb amputation.

Determining if someone has capacity to consent / is competent

Before you can obtain consent from a patient, you must ensure that they are competent, i.e. that they have the capacity to make the decision to go ahead with the proposed treatment or procedure.

The assessment of mental capacity should be made in accordance with the Mental Capacity Act 2005 (or the Adults with Incapacity Act 2000 in Scotland). Essentially, a patient is considered to have capacity if he:

- Understands the information provided in relation to the decision that needs to be made
- Is able to retain the information
- Is able to use and weigh up the information
- Can communicate his decision, by whatever means possible.

Every adult is presumed to have capacity

English law dictates that every adult should be assumed to have capacity to consent unless proven otherwise. Essentially, this means that the patient retains full control of decisions affecting his care (i.e. his autonomy) unless someone challenges this assumption and conclusively proves otherwise.

A seemingly irrational decision does not imply lack of capacity

If a patient makes a decision that you consider irrational (such as refuses life-saving treatment), it does not mean that they lack capacity. Similarly, you should not presume that someone is incompetent because they have a mental illness, are too young, can't communicate easily, have beliefs that go against yours or make decisions with which you disagree.

If you are unsure about your assessment

There may be situations where you are unsure as to whether a patient should be considered to have capacity to consent or not. In such cases, you should:

- Ask the nursing staff who know the patient about their ability to make decisions

- Involve colleagues with more specialist knowledge such as a psychiatrist or a neurologist

Some hospitals have a clinical ethics team who can consider the particulars of the case and advise. If you are still unsure you should seek legal advice as a court may need to make that decision.

11.4 | Seeking informed consent from a competent patient

Definition of informed consent

Informed consent is the agreement, granted by a patient, to receive a given treatment, or have a specified procedure performed on them, in full consideration of the facts and implications. The following sections summarise the key issues that you need to be aware of for your interview.

Basic model to obtain informed consent from competent patients

When the patient is competent, seeking informed consent is a relatively straightforward process, as follows:

Step 1: The patient and the doctor discuss the presenting complaint. During the consultation, the doctor gauges the level of understanding of the patient, takes account of their views and values, and presents a range of possible management options.

Step 2: The doctor describes the available options, including:
- Diagnosis and prognosis, including degree of certainty and further investigations required
- Different management options available to the patient, including the outcome of receiving no treatment. It is likely that the doctor will recommend a preferred course of action, but he should in no circumstances coerce the patient
- Details of any necessary investigations/treatments and/or procedures, including their purpose, their nature and which professionals will be involved
- Details of the risks, benefits, side-effects and likelihood of success. The doctor should inform the patient of any serious possible risks (e.g. death, paralysis, etc.) even if the likelihood of occurrence is very small. He should also inform the patient about less serious side-effects or complications if they occur frequently
- Whether the procedure or treatment is part of a research programme or innovative treatment, as well as their right to refuse to participate in research or teaching projects
- Their right to a second opinion.
- Any treatment which you or your Trust cannot provide, but which may be of greater benefit to the patient. This may include procedures for which no one has been trained in your hospital, or treatments not provided by your trust on grounds of cost, but which may be provided elsewhere.

The information should be provided using terms that the patient can understand and the doctor should check the understanding of the patient, answering the patient's questions as appropriate. When asked questions, the doctor should endeavour to respond in the most informative manner, avoiding coercion. If necessary, the doctor should use all necessary means of communication, including visual aids, leaflets, and models.

Step 3   The patient weighs up the benefits and risks and determines whether to accept or refuse the proposed options. If the patient refuses, then the doctor should explore their reasons and continue the discussion as long as the patient wants to. There may be concerns which were not identified or addressed previously. The doctor should inform the patient that they have the right to a second opinion and the opportunity to change their mind later on, if they so wish.

There are circumstances when further procedures may be necessary during the primary planned procedure (e.g. blood transfusion, or doing a different surgical procedure). You need to explain these anticipated risks to the patient clearly and obtain consent for these potential procedures (otherwise you will need to wake the patient up to seek further consent).

Who should seek consent from the patient?

The responsibility to seek consent from the patient rests with the doctor who is proposing the treatment or will be carrying out the procedure. It is possible to delegate the task to someone else, but only if the person seeking the consent is suitably trained and qualified and they have appropriate knowledge of the treatment/procedure and the associated risks. Although the task of consenting is delegated, the responsibility still rests with the doctor who is proposing the treatment or doing the procedure.

Verbal v. written consent

The importance of recording consent is to demonstrate that the process took place with due care and diligence and that both parties had a shared vision of the proposed procedure and any key complications.

In many cases, implied or verbal consent is sufficient. For example, if a patient undresses so that you can examine them, their compliance constitutes consent.

For simple or routine procedures, investigations or treatment, verbal consent may be sufficient. However, you must make sure that the patient has properly understood the information provided and has taken an informed decision. You should also ensure that their consent is duly recorded in their notes, together with the information on which it was based.

You should get written consent:
- For complex or more involved procedures
- If there are serious risks involved
- If there are potential consequences for the patient's employment, social or personal life
- When providing clinical care is not the primary purpose of the investigation or procedure
- When the treatment is part of a research or innovative programme
- For procedures where written consent is required by law (such as organ donation or fertility treatment).

11.5 Dealing with a patient who lacks capacity

When a patient lacks capacity, the doctor must provide care which is in the patient's best interest. It is preferable for the patient to be as involved as they can be in any discussion about their care.

Whatever decisions are being taken by the doctor, the patient should be treated with respect, dignity and should not be discriminated against. In making decisions on behalf of the patient, the doctor should take account of a wide range of issues, including:

- Whether the patient has signed an advance directive stating how he wants to be treated in situations when he can't give informed consent

- The views of any individuals who are legally representing the patient or whom the patient has said they wanted to involve

- The views of any individuals who are close to the patient and may be able to comment on their beliefs, values and feelings (e.g. their relatives)

- Whether the lack of capacity is temporary (e.g. the patient may be temporarily unconscious) or permanent.

Unless the patient has signed an advance directive, the management decisions will rest with the doctor. Legally, relatives and others only have an advisory role. In practice, the doctor should try to seek a consensus around the care of the patient by involving all relevant parties in the discussions.

Sometimes there are disagreements, either between the doctor and the rest of their team, or between the medical team and those close to the patient. In situations such as these, it is important to seek conflict resolution through negotiation. Useful resources could include consulting more experienced colleagues, using mediation services or independent advocates. In cases of more severe disagreements then legal advice should be sought and a court decision may be needed.

11.6 Competence/capacity in children

Can children give informed consent?

All children aged 16 or above can be assumed to be competent, i.e. essentially they can be treated in exactly the same way as an adult. Children under the age of 16 can give consent to a treatment, procedure or investigation if they are deemed to be Gillick competent, in reference to a famous House of Lords ruling on the ability of children under 16 to consent – see 11.7 for details on the Gillick case.

A child is deemed Gillick competent if they can understand, retain, use and weigh the information given and their understanding of benefits, risks and consequences.

Involving the parents

Even if a child is competent enough to make a decision to consent to a given procedure or treatment, you should make every effort to encourage the child to involve their parents. Whatever their involvement, parents cannot override consent given by a competent child.

Can children refuse treatment?

In Scotland, the situation is simple. Children can refuse treatment and the child's decision cannot be overridden by the parents. In England, Wales and Northern Ireland, no minor can refuse consent to treatment, when consent has been given by someone with parental responsibility or by the court. This applies even if the child is competent and specifically refuses treatment that is considered to be in their best interest. This is a rare event and you should seek legal advice through your Trust and your defence union. Enforcing treatment on a child against their will poses risks which need to be weighed up against the benefits of the procedure or treatment. You will also undoubtedly need to involve other members of the multidisciplinary team and an independent advocate for the child.

The above is the essential information that you will be required to know for most interviews. If you are applying for Paediatrics or Obstetrics and Gynaecology, or want further detail on children's consent, you can consult the GMC booklet *0-18 years – guidance for all doctors* online at www.gmc-uk.org.

11.7 Gillick competence & Fraser guidelines

In specialties where children are involved, questions are sometimes asked that require some basic knowledge of Gillick competence and Fraser guidelines.

These two concepts both relate to the ability of children to give consent for treatment, without the need for parental consent or knowledge. However, many candidates misunderstand or confuse the two concepts. In reality, although linked, they are slightly different. The purpose of this section is to explain what they mean and how they differ.

Gillick competence – The House of Lords ruling

In 1980 the Department of Health and Social Services (DHSS) advised doctors that children under the age of 16 could be prescribed contraception, without parental consent.

Mrs Gillick, the mother of ten children including five daughters, sought a declaration from the House of Lords that the DHSS guidance was unlawful and adversely affected parental rights and duties. Her main arguments were that the decision was the same as administering treatment to a child without consent (which should rest with the parents), and that this encouraged others to commit the offence of having sexual relationships with a minor. Although she had won 3:0 in the Court of Appeal, she lost 2:3 in the House of Lords.

In 1985, the House of Lords panel, led by Lord Fraser, ruled that parental rights did not exist and that, if a minor was competent, they could consent to treatment without the parents being able to veto that decision. It was also ruled that the test of competence for minors should be the same as the test for competence for adults. This is now referred to as "Gillick competence". Although the Gillick case was originally solely about contraception, the ruling was general and applies to any treatment, investigation or procedure.

Further ruling

In 1990, a further ruling stated that a "Gillick-competent" child can prevent their parents from viewing their medical records. Consent must be sought explicitly.

Fraser guidelines

Following on from the Gillick case, Lord Fraser released further guidelines specifically relating to contraception (which can also be extended to abortion).

These guidelines state that a doctor or other health professional providing contra-ceptive advice or treatment to someone under 16, without parental consent, should be satisfied that:

- The young person will understand the advice;
- The young person will understand the moral, social and emotional implica-tions;
- The young person cannot be persuaded to tell their parents or allow the doc-tor to tell them that they are seeking contraceptive advice;
- The young person is having, or is likely to have, unprotected sex whether they receive the advice or not;
- Their physical or mental health is likely to suffer unless they receive the ad-vice or treatment; and
- It is in the young person's best interests to give contraceptive advice or treat-ment without parental consent.

11.8 | Mental Capacity Act 2005 (effective 2007)

Although no in-depth knowledge of the Mental Capacity Act 2005 is required, other than perhaps for Psychiatry interviews at ST4 level, candidates will be expected to know its key points. Indeed, candidates in many specialties have been asked what they know of the Mental Capacity Act 2005. Some have been given scenarios where some basic knowledge of the Act was required.

Many of the Mental Capacity Act 2005's provisions have been described in previous sections on consent. This section summarises the key components of the Act.

Purpose of the Act

The Act formalises best practice and common law principles, in relation to the care of patients who lack capacity, and those who make decisions on their behalf.

Assessing lack of capacity

- No one can be assumed to lack capacity simply because they have a specific medical condition.

- Lack of capacity cannot be established in relation to someone's age, appearance or behaviour which may lead others to make assumptions. So, for example:
  - children are not necessarily lacking capacity simply because they are young
  - someone who is unkempt does not necessarily lack capacity simply because they are not looking after themselves
  - Someone behaving eccentrically or making decisions which appear unusual or counter-intuitive does not necessarily lack capacity.

- Any action or decision taken on behalf of someone who lacks capacity must be taken in their best interest. Best interest can be assessed by asking the patient to write their wishes down (e.g. advanced directive) and by consulting those who are familiar with the patient, e.g. relatives or carers.

- Anyone providing care to a person who lacks capacity can do so without the risk of incurring legal liability, provided that capacity has been properly assessed and that care is being provided in line with the patient's best interest.

- The use or threat of force (called "restraint") is only permitted if the person using it believes that it will prevent harm to the patient who lacks capacity.

Making decisions on behalf of an incapable patient & legal framework

- A patient with capacity is allowed to appoint an attorney to make health and welfare decisions on their behalf, should they ever lose capacity. This is called "Lasting Powers of Attorney" (LPA).

- Deputies may be appointed by the courts to make decisions in relation to welfare, healthcare and finances, though they cannot refuse consent to life-sustaining treatment. These court-appointed deputies will be supervised by the newly-created post of Public Guardian.

- A new Court of Protection has been set up to provide final rulings on matters of capacity.

Protecting vulnerable people

- If a patient lacks capacity, but has no one to speak on their behalf, then an Independent Mental Capacity Advocate (IMCA) can be appointed to represent them. The IMCA cannot make decisions, but represents the patient by bringing to the attention of decision-makers (e.g. doctors) the important factors that need to be considered, such as the patient's beliefs, feelings and values. The IMCA can also challenge decisions on behalf of the patient.

- Advanced decisions to refuse treatment: patients may provide an advanced statement that they refuse to receive treatment should they lose capacity in the future (e.g. DNR orders). The Act states that the advanced decision can only be valid if a proper process has been followed. In particular, the statement must be in writing, signed and witnessed. For an advanced statement to be valid in cases of life-threatening events, the document must state explicitly that it is valid "even if life is at risk".

Using incapable patients in research (this section would be relevant for those applying to academic posts)

- Any research involving patients lacking capacity should be approved by a Research Ethics Committee. One condition is that there is no other alternative, i.e. that the research cannot be carried out using patients who have capacity instead.

- Approval should be sought from carers or nominated third parties before the patient can participate in the research. In particular, they should make a judgement as to whether the patient would have wanted to be involved.

If the patient concerned refuses to be involved or shows any sign of resistance, then they should not be included.

11.9   Consent when dealing with emergencies in the clinical setting

If you are dealing with emergencies in the clinical setting, then all the rules described in previous sections apply.

If a patient is competent at that time and needs a procedure, you should seek consent, even if only verbal.

If the patient is not competent and you cannot determine the patient's wishes through the relatives or other sources, then you can treat them without their consent, on the condition that the treatment that you administer is limited to what is immediately necessary to save their life or prevent a serious deterioration of their condition. The guidelines also specify that the treatment you provide must be the least restrictive of the patient's future choices. If the patient regains capacity, you should explain what was done. For any other treatment beyond the strict minimum, you should seek consent from the patient.

For children, the same applies. The guidance issued by the GMC in *0-18 years: guidance for all doctors*[10] states that "you can provide emergency treatment without consent to save the life of, or prevent serious deterioration in the health of, a child or young person". Of course, this does not preclude you from involving the parents. If the parents disagreed with your emergency treatment, then you would be entitled to proceed with what you perceived to be in the best interest of the child.

---

[10] www.gmc-uk.org/guidance/ethical_guidance/children_guidance_index.asp

11.10 Dealing with emergencies outside the clinical setting

Occasionally questions are asked about the behaviour you should adopt if an emergency takes place outside the clinical setting (e.g. you are on a plane or on holiday).

Do you have to get involved?

To answer this question, there are two principles to consider:

GMC guideline (Good Medical Practice 2013, article 26)
This describes your medical responsibility as a doctor as: "You must offer help if emergencies arise in clinical settings or in the community, taking account of your own safety, your competence and the availability of other options for care."

Essentially this means that, providing you are safe (e.g. not in the middle of a busy motorway or under physical threat by someone) and providing you will not make things worse, then you are obliged to help.

Situations where a doctor may not be competent to help would include someone who has been out of clinical practice for a long time and may actually harm the patient by intervening directly. In that situation they should ensure that the right people are called. In an emergency in a completely different specialty, the patient may be better off being sent to hospital straight away, rather than being treated on site.

You need to make a judgement based on the circumstances. If you are in the middle of the jungle, there is no way the patient will ever get to a hospital, and the only alternative is death, their best bet may be you, even if you feel shaky in your knowledge. Essentially you must weigh up the different options and ensure that you choose the alternative which is best for the patient.

The law
In the UK, unlike the US, there is no specific "Good Samaritan" law. In fact, under UK law, there is no obligation for anyone (including a doctor) to assist another human who needs resuscitation or emergency assistance, unless that person has caused the problem in the first place.

Therefore, from a legal perspective you can choose to ignore an emergency if you wish, BUT from a medical perspective the GMC will require you to get involved as set out in the previous paragraph. If you refuse to get involved or choose to ignore the matter, you won't be sued, but you would be in breach of the GMC's duties of a doctor and may be reported to the GMC if this is discovered.

What if you do get involved and it goes wrong?

As soon as you get involved with an emergency outside the clinical setting, then you have a duty of care towards the patient and must act in their best interest. This means that you may be legally liable if your intervention leaves the patient in a worse position than if you had not intervened.

If the alternative for the patient was death (e.g. if he was arresting), then there is no problem; any action is better than no action providing it is in line with what would be expected in those circumstances. However, if the patient is not in danger of death you must think carefully about your actions to ensure that the patient does not come to more harm, than if no action had been taken.

11.11　Reading list

For the most part, issues of consent and confidentiality are often common sense. There is little that you actually need to memorise once you have read this chapter, understood how these concepts interact and how they may apply in your clinical practice.

In an interview, when questions are asked that relate to consent and confidentiality, the interviewers will expect you to demonstrate a degree of confidence and fluency. They will also expect you to demonstrate that you can involve the appropriate colleagues and other sources of help if you do not know the answer to the question. The information contained in this chapter will be more than enough for any interview at CT or ST level.

Available from the GMC website (www.gmc-uk.org)

- *Consent: patients and doctors making decisions together* (2008)[11]
- *0-18 years: guidance for all doctors*[12]
- *Confidentiality* (2009)[13]

All three documents are written in lay language and can be read quickly.

Available from the Office of Public Sector Information

- Mental Capacity Act 2005[14]

  This document is complex to read (legal jargon and with a formal legal format) so I would recommend that you read it only if you have an interest in these issues and a few hours to spare! Otherwise the summary provided in section 11.8 will be more than enough.

---

[11] www.gmc-uk.org/guidance/ethical_guidance/consent_guidance_index.asp
[12] www.gmc-uk.org/guidance/ethical_guidance/children_guidance_index.asp
[13] www.gmc-uk.org/guidance/ethical_guidance/confidentiality.asp
[14] www.opsi.gov.uk/ACTS/acts2005/ukpga_20050009_en_1

12 Difficult scenarios

Questions relating to confidentiality, consent or other ethical issues can be asked at interviews in any specialties.

Cascading questions

When ethical, consent and confidentiality issues are tested in the form of verbal interview questions (as opposed to role play), they tend to be asked in a cascading fashion, i.e. you are asked a simple initial question and, as soon as you provide an answer, the interviewers tell you that your approach is not working and add extra information to make the problem more complex.

For example, you explain that you deal with a problem by seeking help from a Registrar; the interviewers will tell you that he is not available. You then state that you would contact the consultant on call. The interviewers tell you that he is not answering his phone; and so on. The best way you can deal with them is by:

- Remaining calm and remembering that these questions are not designed to make you fail but to test your understanding of the issues involved
- Making sure that you do not simply explain what you would do, but how you arrive at that conclusion, i.e. what is driving your actions, explaining the ethical principles that you use whenever appropriate
- Reassuring yourself that what is important is your thinking process, so make sure that you set out the logic of your arguments.

Once you have learnt to deal with a few key scenarios, then you can pretty much deal with any scenario which is thrown at you. Therefore, instead of learning all possible scenarios by heart, make sure that you understand the basic concepts which underpin the management of each situation. The theory set out in Section 11 and the examples that follow should help you with this.

All scenarios set out in this section are actual scenarios asked at CT and ST interviews. For each scenario, I have also shown appropriate probing questions.

12.1   <u>Medical specialties</u>: **You have a 20-year-old patient on the ward. She has told you that she does not get on with her father and that, if he calls, you should not tell him anything about her condition. Later on that day, one of the nurses tells you that the father is on the phone, aggressively demanding some information. What do you do?**

The ethics

In normal circumstances, most patients would authorise you to provide information to their relatives. In this case, however, the patient has explicitly told you that she did not want her father to be told anything and therefore you have to respect her wishes.

The fact that the patient is 20 years old is in fact a red herring because the same principle would apply to a 14-year-old. In principle, every patient is entitled to confidentiality unless you have a good reason to breach it.

The communication

From an ethical point of view, the answer is almost too simple. What the interviewers will therefore be more interested in is the way in which you handle the matter. There are dozens of ways in which this can be achieved; here are some:

- Ask the nurse to reassure the father that someone will be with him shortly. If it may be some time, the father should be told that someone will call back shortly.
- Use the time to discuss with the daughter whether she stands by her decision. You may want to enquire as to the reasons behind her refusal to see if there is an easy way of breaking the deadlock. You should not push too far (you don't want to be involved too much in their family feuds).
- See if you can try to reach a compromise. For example, if the patient is not in any danger, she may agree to her father being told that she is fine so that he is reassured (after all, he may not be concerned about the detail of the problem and simply wants to know that his daughter is safe).
- Take the phone call (or call the father back) and introduce yourself.
- Provide the father with whatever information was agreed with the patient. If the patient asked you to say nothing at all, then you will need to explain this to the father sensitively.
- Recommend that the father talks to his daughter directly.
- If the father insists or becomes more aggressive, explain that you will discuss the matter with a senior colleague and hang up after the usual civilities.
- Discuss the matter with a consultant.

Probing: Still unhappy, the father turns up on the ward that afternoon demanding an explanation. He is abusive towards members of staff. What do you do?

Your priority will be the safety of the staff, the patient and the other patients. You and suitable staff members should take the father away from the ward. If he causes problems, you should call the security team.

Once the father has been isolated, you should make sure that no one is on their own with him. Take a colleague with you and talk to him about the situation. The father should be reminded that his behaviour is not acceptable, after which you should determine what his causes for worry are.

Similar principles to the telephone conversation will apply from then on, i.e. you can only reveal information which has been agreed with the patient. If the father wants to know more, then you should encourage him to discuss the matter with his daughter.

When the father has left, you may want to discuss the matter further with the daughter to see if you can break the deadlock.

12.2   <u>Surgical specialties</u>: **You are on call at night. A patient is brought to you as an emergency. The patient requires a specific procedure that you have never done before. You have only observed a consultant once for this procedure. If the procedure is not carried out soon the patient will suffer serious harm. What do you do?**

This is a question which is very common in surgical interviews. At the actual interview, the procedure in question will be named (but it will always be something that you will have little experience of) and the harm to the patient will also be specified (e.g. loss of limb).

The initial answer to the question is not actually that difficult, but most candidates fall down at the probing stage. Keep calm and think logically.

Answer:
- Make sure that the patient is stabilised and taken to theatre as soon as possible.
- Call for help from a senior colleague on site (anyone who can perform the procedure in question). If none is available, then call for a senior on call.

Probing: Your Registrar is dealing with another emergency and cannot come. The only other person available is the consultant on call. However, you cannot reach him. His phone seems to be turned off.

Answer:
- Call another consultant, even if they are not on call.

Probing: The only other consultant available is at a party and tells you that he is too drunk to be safe. He tells you that you should "do what you think is best".

Answer:
- Discuss with the site manager (usually a senior nurse) who may have some useful suggestions.
- See if you can contact a team from another hospital. It is not ideal but it may be your best bet.
- At this point you should really consider seeking additional advice from your defence union's 24-hour helpline (providing you can find the time without harming the patient).

Probing: There is no one else to help you. Essentially you are on your own and you cannot wait much longer before the patient is harmed.

Answer:
- Think about whether you could use the help from the "drunk" consultant. He is obviously not the safest person to deal with the problem, but nor are you. He may be drunk but he may still be able to help you out by giving you directions to deal with the procedure. You can only consider this alternative if you feel that it is safer than (i) doing the procedure by yourself and (ii) doing nothing.
- If the consultant is not able to help or if he refuses, then you will need to weigh up the two options left to you: (i) do it yourself or (ii) do nothing; and choose the option which will cause the least harm to the patient.

The "least unsafe" principle

There is no way to deal with the situation in a safe manner since the interviewers are constantly placing hurdles in your way to make it as unsafe as they can. In this scenario, none of the safe options are available to you and therefore you must opt for the least unsafe solution.

In some cases, if the choice is between "having a go" and "death", then there is nothing to lose by having a go providing you feel that there is a chance that you might succeed. It is all about balancing benefits against risks.

Risk management

Once the situation is over, you must then deal with the other issues. In this scenario there are a few issues that need to be addressed with the team:

- The unavailability of the consultant on call.
- The lack of help from the drunken consultant. He should have helped you find suitable alternatives at least. The fact that the consultant is drunk should not be cause for concern in terms of his integrity, since he is not on call.
- You will most likely need to complete a critical incident form.

12.3   <u>Medical specialties</u>: **One of your patients is refusing to adhere to your recommended treatment. As a result, her condition is deteriorating rapidly. What do you do?**

At an interview, the interviewers may specify the condition in question, the recommended treatment and the level of deterioration. Although some of the clinical management will differ depending on the specific information given, the main issues will remain the same. The danger with this question is to spend too much time dealing with the clinical side and not enough dealing with the other needs of the patient and the ethical issues at stake.

Answer:
- The patient has a right of autonomy, i.e. if she wants to refuse the treatment that you feel is best for her, then she can and you should respect her decision.

- However, you would not be acting in the patient's best interest (i.e. you would breach your duty of beneficence) if you allowed her to make that decision without ensuring she has fully understood the consequences and without making sure that she is aware of possible alternatives.

- Enquire with the patient about the reasons for her refusal to adhere to treatment and determine whether there are easy ways of solving the problem.
    - Physical reasons: does the patient suffer from unwanted side-effects? Does the patient have an issue with the method of delivery (tablets, injections, etc.)? Perhaps these are easily addressed by adopting a different treatment or providing additional help (e.g. further medication).
    - Psychological reasons: does the patient experience negative feelings or depression? If this is the case then she may need to be referred to a counsellor. Does the patient find it difficult to remember to take her medication?
    - Social reasons: does the patient have a lifestyle which is incompatible with the treatment? Does the medication interfere in any way with her lifestyle? A discussion with the patient or a change of regimen may address the problem.

Throughout your discussions with the patient, make sure that you inform the patient without coercing her (otherwise you may harm her trust in you and you would also go against her right to autonomy).

- Educate the patient on the consequences of not taking the medication. You need to make sure that the decision she is making is informed. Your duty of beneficence dictates that you must act in the best interest of the patient.

- Propose appropriate action, depending on the needs identified earlier, and provide the patient with further information (e.g. leaflets).
- If the patient feels that she needs time to consider the options, allow that time. You may also suggest that she consults with relatives, or offer to talk to them yourself if you can get the patient's agreement (so as not to breach confidentiality).

- Organise a review of the patient at a suitable interval to monitor progress.

- All of this makes the assumption that the patient is competent. The fact that the patient is making an irrational decision does not mean that she is not competent. However, if you suspect that she may not have capacity to consent then you should seek senior advice and/or assessment by a psychiatrist.

Probing: What would you do if the patient was lacking capacity?

Answer:
- You would need to consult your team to determine the best way forward.

- You would need to determine whether the lack of capacity is temporary or permanent. If it is temporary then you may be able to wait until the patient gains her capacity again.

- With a patient who lacks capacity, it falls back onto the doctor to act in the best interest of the patient. You would need to involve her relatives or carers in discussions if appropriate.

- It may be difficult to administer a treatment against the patient's will, so you should continue to discuss with the patient to try to get them to consent.

Probing: Assume that the patient has full capacity. She is still refusing treatment. What next?

Answer:
- If the patient refuses consent whilst having full capacity then there is absolutely nothing you can do other than accept her decision.

- However, you would still need to act in her best interest as far as you can, for example by offering pain-reduction solutions or palliative options.

- You may also offer a regular follow-up to the patient.

12.4	<u>Surgical specialties</u>: **An adult is brought into A&E. He is unconscious, bleeding profusely and may require a blood transfusion. The accompanying relatives tell you that the patient is a long-standing Jehovah's Witness. What do you do?**

This scenario is almost a viva question for a surgical exam and ranks high in terms of difficulty. I would say that it is well above what most candidates should expect to get at their interview. Nevertheless, it was asked at several ST3 surgical interviews and, as a result, I felt that it was important to include it in this book to stretch the more ambitious candidates.

The underlying problem

A Jehovah's Witness would refuse a blood transfusion. However, we are only being told that the patient is a Jehovah's Witness. Unfortunately the patient is unconscious and therefore cannot give consent or express his wishes.

In such a situation, you have to act in the best interest of the patient which, in this case, means doing what the patient would have wanted you to do if he had been able to give consent. The problem is: "How do you establish what he would have wanted?"

Patient safety & first-line solution

In the first instance you will need to organise for the patient to be made safe by whatever clinical means are appropriate (theatre, etc.). You would also need to call your Registrar or your consultant as soon as possible. If they are not around then anyone senior who can help with the discussions will do.

There are also questions that you need to ask yourself:

- If blood transfusion is a problem, are you able to use blood-free alternatives? This would solve the problem.
- Is there a possibility that the emergency can be dealt with without a blood transfusion at all (the question says that the patient "may" require one)?
- Can you delay the need for a transfusion until more information is gathered (e.g. by giving plasma expanders)?

Probing: There are no blood-free alternatives and the patient will need a transfusion. What do you do?

Simultaneously to all this, investigations into the patient's background should take place:

- Does the patient carry a card on them indicating that they are a Jehovah's Witness and would not consent to a blood transfusion?
- Has the patient got notes at the hospital which would confirm the position (for example, they might have refused a transfusion on a previous occasion when they were competent)?
- Is there dissent amongst the relatives about the patient's position (in case of dissent, you would be more inclined to opt for the blood transfusion than not).

The answers to these questions may help you determine the patient's wishes. You should of course ensure that your seniors are involved (even if this means waking them up in the middle of the night). There may also be a need to involve the medical director or anyone who holds high-level responsibilities as there may be a legal issue. You should also ensure that the family is fully involved so that their views can be clarified.

If there is time, you could try to obtain a court order. At the very least you should get legal advice from your medical defence union's 24-hour helpline to drive your decision making.

Probing: Despite all this, you cannot obtain enough information to determine the patient's wishes and no one is around to help you. What do you do?

If you really have no idea as to what to do, it is always best to opt for what <u>you</u> regard as being the best option. In this case, this would mean transfusing the patient. If this is the case, then you must ensure that you document exactly what has happened.

Keep in touch with your medical defence union. This is important because the patient may then object to your actions and may take subsequent action against you or the Trust. You must therefore be in a position to back up your behaviour fully if the case came to court. Having said that, it would be easier to justify keeping someone alive than letting them die if there was no certainty at all.

Probing: What if the patient is in fact an unconscious child and the parents are refusing a blood transfusion on his behalf?

The guidelines are that, in an emergency, you can treat a child without consent. However, you should try to involve the parents if you can, either by allowing them to change their mind or by discussing the use of blood-free alternatives if it is a safe compromise and would achieve similar results to blood transfusion (i.e. if this did not go against the child's best interest).

As much as possible, you should not take such a decision by yourself and you should involve suitable senior colleagues. There will be a specific local policy. You should also keep in touch with your medical defence union.

If blood alternatives are not available, or there is no way to avoid a transfusion, then you would be entitled to proceed with a transfusion.

If there is time (administering plasma expanders may have allowed you that time) and it is practical to do so, you should try to get a court order. It goes without saying that everything should be duly documented.

Here is the advice from the GMC:

Refusal of blood products by Jehovah's Witnesses

Many Jehovah's Witnesses have strong objections to the use of blood and blood products, and may refuse them, even if there is a possibility that they may die as a result.

You should not make assumptions about the decisions that a Jehovah's Witness patient might make about treatment with blood or blood products. You should ask for and respect their views and answer their questions honestly and to the best of your ability. You may also wish to contact the hospital liaison committees established by the Watchtower Society (the governing body of Jehovah's Witnesses) to support Jehovah's Witnesses faced with treatment decisions involving blood. These committees can advise on current Society policy regarding the acceptability or otherwise of particular blood products. They also keep details of hospitals and doctors who are experienced in "bloodless" medical procedures.

www.gmc-uk.org/guidance/ethical_guidance/personal_beliefs/personal_beliefs.asp

12.5   <u>O&G</u>: A 14-year-old girl mentions that she is pregnant and enquires about an abortion. What do you do?

- The girl is 14 years old. According to the Gillick competence principle and Fraser guidelines, if she is competent then she would be able to consent to an abortion. You would then need to assess her competence, which could be done through a simple discussion. In accordance with the Fraser guidelines, you will need to discuss with the patient the need to involve the parents, though you cannot enforce it if she refuses. She may benefit from parental involvement if she requires support after the procedure.

- Confirm that she is indeed pregnant. If she is, then you need to enquire about the circumstances of the pregnancy, if your relationship with the patient makes this possible. Not only will this enable you to identify whether there are any issues relating to child abuse, but you may also be able to use this discussion to discuss contraception, sexual health and other related issues. The circumstances are likely to have a psychological impact on the young person in which case you may wish to offer counselling.

- You should discuss the case with some of your colleagues to determine whether there is cause for concern in relation to her age. If necessary, you may need to breach confidentiality by raising the matter with social services, or other appropriate organisations. This decision will need to be taken with your team, and you ought to discuss it with the patient first.

- Your success will depend on your verbal and non-verbal communication skills during the consultation. Ensure that your approach is non-judgemental, empathic and conducive to establishing a good rapport in order to develop and maintain trust.

- If the child is not Gillick competent then you would require the parents' consent. If the child refuses to allow you to divulge information to her parents about her case, then you would need to convince her to accept to be represented by an appropriate person. If she refuses, then, provided that you deem the abortion to be in the best interest of the child, in theory you would be entitled to proceed with the abortion. However, given the complexity of the situation, you would need to discuss with your team and possibly even need a court order.

12.6	**All**: You are a Registrar. A young female trainee doctor refuses to deal with a patient who is a known rapist. What do you do?

This question was first asked at Emergency Medicine Registrar interviews but has also appeared in Psychiatry and several other specialties. In such questions it is very easy to jump to conclusions and to assume that the trainee is in breach of her duties by not giving the patient the care he is entitled to. However, the situation may be more complex than it first appears.

You can answer this question using the SPIES structure set out in section 5.3.

Seek information
Although you would want to find out more about the reasons behind the trainee's decision, the time for discussion will come later once the immediate issue of patient care/safety has been dealt with.

Patient care/safety
The patient is entitled to care, regardless of his background, and you must ensure that it is delivered by someone whose behaviour is not being affected by their beliefs.

There may be several reasons for the trainee to refuse to see the patient and this will need to be investigated. Whether she feels threatened in any way or whether it is simply on principle, she is not best placed to treat this particular patient (after all, there is no point forcing her). Therefore you may want to manage the patient yourself or to delegate the responsibility to someone who is more willing.

Initiative
Once the patient's problem has been resolved, you ought to organise a discussion with the junior trainee to get to the bottom of the issue as her behaviour may have consequences on the future delivery of patient care, particularly if there are other types of patients that she finds it difficult to deal with. You will want to identify why she refused to manage the patient.

- Perhaps she or someone close to her was raped in the past. If this were the case, she may feel physically threatened (even if there was no explicit threat from the patient) and would not be safe in dealing with the patient.
- Perhaps the patient actually made some remarks towards her, in which case she might have felt physically threatened.
- Perhaps she is simply prejudiced and is making a point of principle. If this were the case, she would likely be in breach of her duties as a doctor, which requires that doctors should not let their personal beliefs interfere with the care of patients.

If the trainee had felt threatened, then she would need support from a senior colleague to overcome such fears and agree a strategy, should the problem occur again.

If the trainee showed signs of prejudice then you would need to remind her of her duties and would also need to report the matter to a senior colleague so that they can discuss the situation with her.

Escalate

Either way this looks like a serious situation, which could have serious effects on the trainee's mental wellbeing. Whether there has been a breach of duty or not, it would make sense to encourage the trainee to discuss the matter with a senior colleague, and, if this does not happen, to raise the matter yourself albeit informally.

There is also a chance that the patient may make a complaint and it would make sense for senior colleagues to be made aware of the problem before the patient himself escalates it.

Support

Whichever way you look at the situation, the trainee has clearly been affected by the matter and you owe her a degree of support. In some circumstances (e.g. if the question is being asked in a Psychiatry interview) it may also be wise to question the trainee's career choice, and perhaps to encourage her to think more rationally about future career plans.

If there were a number of members of staff affected by this patient or incident, it may be worth organising a team debrief, facilitated by an appropriate professional, such as a psychologist.

12.7 All: You find out that one of your consultants is romantically involved with someone who is a current patient of the department. What do you do?

This question is difficult because, although we are told that the patient is a current patient of the department, it is not clear whether that patient is being treated by that consultant. It is possible that the consultant in question told his/her partner to get referred to their own department because they have faith in the quality of the service being delivered there, thinking it would be fine if they are not themselves seeing their own partner in clinic.

The whole answer rests on the notion of whether this would seem appropriate or not, and this is not always clear-cut.

Scenario 1 – The consultant is treating the patient (or involved in some way in the patient's care).

This situation is inappropriate. If the relationship started before the partner became a patient, then the partner should not be treated by the consultant. If the relationship started when the partner was already a patient, then this is even more improper.

The matter should be reported to the consultant's line manager (i.e. the clinical director), and the GMC would then likely be notified.

Scenario 2 – The consultant is not treating the patient (or involved in any way in the patient's care)

This situation is a bit more complicated because there is no established doctor-patient relationship as such. However, there are grounds to argue that this can be contentious. For example:

- The consultant has easy access to the partner's medical records.
- The consultant may come across details of the partner's medical condition in settings such as MDT meetings.
- The consultant may influence their colleagues on choice of treatment.

In the interest of transparency, the consultant should be advised to declare their relationship with the patient to their manager (i.e. the clinical director), so that the situation can be discussed, and a conclusion can be reached. In such situation, it is unlikely that the GMC will be involved, but safeguards may be introduced to ensure complete separation between the consultant and the partner's medical records.

What the GMC says

1 - Article 53 of Good Medical Practice states that "You must not use your professional position to pursue a sexual or improper emotional relationship with a patient or someone close to them."

2 - Trust is the foundation of the doctor-patient partnership. Patients should be able to trust that their doctor will behave professionally towards them during consultations and not see them as a potential sexual partner.

Current patients

3 - You must not pursue a sexual or improper emotional relationship with a current patient.

4 - If a patient pursues a sexual or improper emotional relationship with you, you should treat them politely and considerately and try to re-establish a professional boundary. If trust has broken down and you find it necessary to end the professional relationship, you must follow the guidance in 'Ending your professional relationship with a patient'.

5 - You must not use your professional relationship with a patient to pursue a relationship with someone close to them. For example, you must not use home visits to pursue a relationship with a member of a patient's family.

6 - You must not end a professional relationship with a patient solely to pursue a personal relationship with them.

Former patients

7 - Personal relationships with former patients may also be inappropriate depending on factors such as:

- the length of time since the professional relationship ended (the more recently a professional relationship with a patient ended, the less likely it is that beginning a personal relationship with that patient would be appropriate).

- the nature of the previous professional relationship.

- whether the patient was particularly vulnerable at the time of the professional relationship, and whether they are still vulnerable.

- whether you will be caring for other members of the patient's family.

12.8 | <u>All specialties</u>: You have been working 13 hours and are about to leave. You feel very tired after a busy shift. The colleague who is taking over from you is late and you are being called to review a patient in A&E. You can see straight away that the matter will take some time to resolve. What do you do?

The European Working Time Directive (EWTD)

Some candidates get very flustered at the thought of having to breach the requirements of the European Working Time Directive. In practice, though, patient safety is far more important than breaching the directive requirements by an hour. In court, you would find it really difficult to justify having let a patient die simply because you had to work an hour on top of requirements. Generally speaking, it is acceptable to breach the EWTD requirements in exceptional circumstances, provided that you receive compensation for it at a later stage. Therefore you do not have to worry about the regulations in this scenario where a patient needs you.

Patient safety

Of greater concern to you will be patient safety. The scenario clearly states that you are feeling very tired. If you feel that you can safely deal with the matter in hand then you should do so. But if you feel that you are struggling because it is the end of your long shift, then you ought to seek help from another colleague. If there is no other colleague available then you will have to get started and organise for someone to take over from you shortly. With a bit of luck your colleague will arrive soon and you won't have to work long. If you cannot get hold of your colleague to get an idea of how long he will be, you need to call your registrar or consultant so that they are aware of the issue and can come in and help if need be. If you have any doubt about your ability to cope or if you see that you may have to stay beyond your threshold for being safe, call your seniors anyway: better to be safe than sorry.

The late colleague

After the event, you will need to address your colleague's lateness. In this particular event it may have led to patient harm (since, despite being tired, you had to handle the situation yourself). If there was no valid excuse or if it happened again, you would need to raise the issue more formally with a senior colleague.

13 NHS issues and hot topics

Most candidates have limited knowledge of NHS structures and policy; as a result, many worry that they could face difficult factual questions which they would be unable to answer.

On the whole, questions on NHS issues are designed to test your general understanding of the issues rather than detailed knowledge of any particular topic. In other words, you are more likely to be asked "How do you feel the specialty will be affected by current NHS changes?" than "Tell us everything you know about the Darzi report". You should therefore make some effort to familiarise yourself with key issues likely to affect the specialty to which you are applying and reflect on their significance to your career and your specialty. By demonstrating a good understanding of these issues, you will present yourself as a mature candidate with strong motivation.

Different types of questions

NHS issues can be tested at interview in three main ways:

- Knowledge questions about a specific topic, e.g. "What is the role of the Care Quality Commission?"

- Awareness questions such as "What do you think about the increasing role of the private sector?"

- Application questions, i.e. questions which require putting together a range of ideas such as "What are the issues affecting this specialty at the moment?" or "How do you see this specialty evolving over the next 5 or 10 years?"

As well as being tested through standard interview questions, your knowledge of NHS issues can be tested through presentations and group discussions.

What the interviewers are looking for

The interviewers will be looking for three features:

- The effort that you have put into keeping abreast of current developments relevant to your specialty, and therefore your motivation for the specialty.

- Your ability to analyse the impact of these issues on your work environment and the health system in general, and therefore your debating ability and general level of maturity.

- Your ability to communicate your ideas in a structured and convincing fashion.

Specialty-specific NHS issues and hot topics

In some interviews, you may be asked about specific documents or issues relating to your specialty. This could include National Service Frameworks (NSFs) and specific NICE or other guidelines. To ensure that you can answer all these questions, you should consult the following sources of information:

- The NHS website for NSFs[15]
- The NICE website[16]
- The relevant Royal College's website[17]

You should ask some of your senior colleagues to point you in the direction of specialty-specific issues and guidelines that are topical at the time of your interview. You should also read specialty-specific papers as interviewers sometimes ask questions on papers that have recently been published.

General NHS issues and hot topics

These are general topics that apply to most specialties. This includes issues such as the current NHS drive towards better quality and more efficiency, the issues of patient choice and increased competition, or issues relating to the impact of current reforms on medical training. It is crucial that you understand the key messages and are able to present your own opinion of the possible impact on the department to which you are applying. It is important to be aware that most reports have a brief Executive Summary that gives the highlights and is easier to digest if you're short of time.

This book contains details of the major issues and institutions which you may be asked about. All these issues have been raised at ST interviews in the past or are current major topics so make sure that you are familiar with them.

A sensible word of advice

In the whole scheme of things, questions on NHS issues do not get asked at many interviews. Having surveyed post-interview junior doctors who attended ISC Medical's courses, fewer than 10% of candidates had been asked questions requiring

---

[15] http://www.nhs.uk/nhsengland/NSF/pages/Nationalserviceframeworks.aspx
[16] http://www.nice.org.uk/
[17] See Chapter 19

any specific knowledge of current topics. These had been asked mainly at ST3/ST4 interviews (though there had been a few exceptions, with some Ophthalmology ST1 interviews containing questions on the threat that Independent Sector Treatment Centres may represent, for example).

In the course of your preparation, although it is important that you gain an overview of current issues, beware not to get bogged down with significant detail as this is never probed into. All that will be required of you is an overall understanding of these issues; the summaries that follow will be more than enough to help you achieve the required level of understanding.

I would advise strongly that you allocate the majority of your preparation time to all the other types of questions addressed in previous chapters – particularly if you are short of time.

13.1 Overview of the NHS in England

Commissioning of services

In England, each hospital essentially operates as an independent business. The decision as to which healthcare provider is allowed to provide which services is made by Clinical Commissioning Groups (CCGs), which consist mainly of local GPs and managers (with a few representatives from hospitals). So, for example, a local CCG may decide that Hospital X should no longer provide hip replacement surgery, because from now on such surgery should be provided by Hospitals Y and Z only.

Legislation that came into effect in 2013 has made it possible for external providers (e.g. charities or even private companies) to offer NHS services. So, for example, a local CCG could decide to award a contract for cataract surgery to a private company rather than to the local hospital (though of course they would need to have a good reason to do that: a good reason being that they feel the private company may provide better quality of care). The process of awarding contracts is known in the NHS as "commissioning".

Because CCGs are local groups and consist mainly of GPs, they cannot commission GP services themselves. Similarly, they can't commission services that need to be provided on a more global scale because of their specialist nature, such as heart and lung transplant surgery or eye cancer care, for two reasons:

1. They don't have the skills and knowledge to understand the exact nature of those services.

2. Those services are provided on a regional or national basis.

Instead, both primary care services and specialist services are commissioned by a higher body, which used to be called the NHS Commissioning Board but is now known simply as NHS England.

Block Contract vs. Payment by Results

Before 2005, hospitals were paid a fixed amount of money every year, designed to cover the cost of healthcare. That system was called "block contract". If a hospital needed more money (i.e. was in deficit compared to their budget), then the government would simply pay more money to that hospital. Conversely if a hospital spent less money (i.e. showed a profit against its budget), then it would have to pay it back to the government. The problem with that approach was that there was no incentive for hospitals to save money or work efficiently.

In 2005, the Labour government introduced the principle of "Payment by Results", whereby a tariff would be set nationally for each clinic and each procedure. Hospitals would no longer receive a fixed amount of money but would instead be paid for each activity they undertook.

So, for example, a hip replacement might have a tariff of £5,000, which would cover the cost of the hospital stay, imaging, the surgery and some follow-up. The amount of the tariff would be set roughly at the average of the cost across all Trusts, meaning that some hospitals would make a loss and others would make a profit. The idea was to encourage those who made a loss to work more efficiently so that they could make a profit and survive.

Pros and cons of Payment by Results

Though there is no doubt that Payment by Results is forcing the NHS to become more efficient, the jury is out as to whether it actually leads to better care. In truth, it is difficult to predict how the situation will evolve, mainly because one needs to give the system a chance to settle before analysing whether the change has been successful. In reality, it is likely that parts of the system will do very well whilst others may struggle to make it work.

At an interview, your concern is simply to demonstrate that you understand the principles and to show an awareness of the main pros and cons. Here are some of the more common positive and negative arguments:

- The tariff is calculated as an average of the actual cost of the procedure or investigation. This means that a number of Trusts will have actual costs below the tariff and will therefore make a profit, whilst other Trusts will have actual costs above the tariff and will therefore make a loss. This will encourage the Trusts that make a loss to become more efficient and may therefore lead to greater cost-efficiency.

- Trusts who find it difficult to become efficient (maybe because they don't do that many cases of a specific type) will need to merge with other Trusts to build economies of scale, or may stop providing some services. This may create local inequalities and increase pressure on service provision in neighbouring places.

- Trusts are paid on the basis of what they code into their IT system. There is therefore a much greater obsession with recording every single activity so that the Trust can be paid accordingly. Also, coding is left to each Trust to carry out. This may lead to abuse (as some departments may be very liberal in their coding). The whole system therefore relies on trust.

- Payment by Results places the emphasis on quantity rather than quality, i.e. the more you work, the more money you get. Although this is a good way to ensure that patients are dealt with quickly (particularly in an environment where waiting time is a common measure of success of the system), it can also be detrimental to patient safety. Action was taken so that hospitals did not just focus on making a profit but also provided quality care to patients. Such actions included:

- Giving patients the choice of where they wanted their care to be provided, whereby the GP would give patients a list of hospitals to which they could go and the patient would then choose the place that suited them most: the hope being that patients would make the choice on the basis of the quality of care they expected to receive.

- Imposing targets that had to be reached (for example, max 4-hour wait in A&E, max 18-week wait for elective surgery).

- Ensuring that hospitals were penalised for poor quality care (for example, by ensuring that, if a patient had to be readmitted to hospital following a complication of the surgery, the hospital would have to deal with that complication without expecting to be paid).

- Introducing incentives to provide enhanced standards of care. For example, the NHS introduced a sort of bonus scheme called CQUIN (Commissioning for Quality and Innovation), which rewards departments that enhance the quality of care of their patients. GPs were encouraged through a sort of bonus scheme too (called QOF – Quality of Outcomes Framework). In addition, hospitals that succeeded in providing best practice care to their patients could benefit from higher tariffs in some specialties.

- Increasing competition between healthcare providers.

- There is controversy about the way in which the tariffs are calculated. Some Trusts argue that their population does not match any kind of national average and the risk that they may lose money is therefore greater than for other Trusts. This can sometimes lead to locally negotiated tariffs to take account of special circumstances.

13.2 The role of the private sector in the provision of healthcare in England

There are several ways in which the private sector is involved and, although you will not need to know any of this in much detail, you must know enough to understand which part of the private sector an interview question is referring to before you can answer it. The different types of private providers are as follows:

1. **Private practice doctors (referred to as "private healthcare"):** this normally refers to doctors working for private hospitals or for themselves who provide healthcare to individual private patients. Examples of private healthcare providers include BUPA or AXA PPP. These private providers have been around for a long time and are normally used by patients to bypass the NHS waiting lists. Patients either pay for the care themselves or through a private healthcare insurance company. The doctors involved in private healthcare are often the same as those working for the NHS, who undertake private activities in their spare time. The prices charged by those private providers are subject to market forces and are typically much higher than the standard NHS tariff for the same procedures.

    So, for example, if a patient has been told that they would need to wait 4 months to get a hip replacement on the NHS but they want it earlier, that patient can go to a private orthopaedic surgeon who will perform the operation a lot sooner. The patient will then have to pay with their own money unless they have private insurance. In exchange they can expect more attention from staff, their own private room and a guarantee to be seen by a consultant.

2. **External (i.e. non-NHS) providers contracted to do NHS work:** this refers to private companies, charities or other organisations who have been officially commissioned to provide healthcare to NHS patients at NHS tariffs. An example of this is Virgin Care who provides services to NHS patients in areas as diverse as breast cancer screening, paediatric physiotherapy, sexual health services or dermatology clinics. Those services are commissioned by the CCGs, and are provided at no direct cost to the patient. Basically this is NHS care provided at NHS tariffs by non-NHS providers.

It is the introduction of those private providers contracted to do NHS work that has led many to fear a "privatisation of the NHS". Here are the arguments commonly presented for and against such a system (which we have tried to present in as balanced a way as possible):

▪ Private companies are run for profit. There is a risk that they will therefore favour making a profit over providing good quality care. The counterargument to this is that the NHS has been run on a not-for-profit basis for many years and has not always provided the best quality care it could (see, later, the section on the Mid-Staffordshire Trust). In addition, though there is some anecdotal evidence that some private companies engage in dubious practices or do not deliver in line with expectations, this is not widespread (and again the NHS has its own share of dubious practices too).

- Private companies may "cherry-pick" the easy cases that are the most profitable, leaving the NHS burdened with the more complex, loss-making cases. The answer to that argument is that it is, indeed, true for the simple reason that one would not want those private companies to take on complex cases they can't handle. Those companies would be asked to handle the simple high volume work to ensure that that work is being done efficiently without interference from other work such as emergencies; it follows then that the NHS (with more expertise than the private sector) should handle the more complex cases that it has been trained to handle well. The reason NHS trusts may be losing money on those more complex cases is because the tariffs have not been calculated well enough to ensure they can cover their costs. However, it is a matter of time before this anomaly is resolved.

- "Privatisation" will lead to fragmentation of care. If different aspects of care are given to different providers then healthcare may be provided in many more venues than under the old system (where basically care was only provided either in a GP practice or in a hospital). This may mean that patients will have to travel to different places in order to be seen, which will cause issues with patient records, for example, since there is no central database that can be accessed from everywhere.

- The fragmentation of care described in the previous paragraph will also lead to training issues. External providers will be handling the simple cases, which are those used as part of medical training. A private company that needs to make a profit may be reluctant to train doctors if that leads to a loss of profit.

- There are risks of conflict of interest amongst doctors. Many of those external providers are, in fact, at least partially owned by doctors. For example, many out-of-hours services are owned by GPs. Some hospital consultants have also set up external businesses, which could be competing against the same hospital trust in which they work. The commissioning of such services therefore has to be done in an open and transparent manner.

13.3   The NHS Long-Term Plan (2019)

Published on 7 January 2019, the NHS Long-Term Plan (formerly known as the 10-year plan) was published, setting out key ambitions for the period 2019-2029. It builds on the previously published NHS Five-Year Forward View, which articulated the needs to integrate care to meet the needs of a changing population. Its main features are as follows:

IMPROVING SERVICES

1 – Clinical priorities

- Key priorities will be cancer, cardiovascular disease (CVD), maternity and neonatal health, mental health, stroke, diabetes and respiratory care. There is also a strong focus on children and young people's health.

- Cancer care: boost survival by speeding up diagnosis, including a package of measures to extend screening and overhaul diagnostic services. New waiting time standards to be introduced requiring patients to get a clear diagnosis for suspected cancer within 28 days of referral by a GP or screening.

- CVD: Improve detection and care for people with CVD and respiratory disease, improve prevention of diabetes and improve stroke services. The aim is to prevent up to 150,000 cases of heart attack, stroke and dementia over the next 10 years.

- Maternity and Neonatal: Aim is to halve the number of still births, maternal mortality, neonatal mortality and serious brain injury in new-born babies by 2025. Measures include: improvement of continuity of care during pregnancy, birth and after-birth; increase in bed capacity in intensive neonatal care and improvement in support from mental health services for pregnant women and new mothers.

2 – Primary and Community Services

- General practices to join together to form primary care networks (essentially groups of neighbouring practices covering 30-50,000 people). These networks will be expected to take a proactive approach to managing population health and will assess the needs of their local population to identify people who would benefit from targeted, proactive support. A shared savings incentivisation scheme will ensure that those networks will benefit financially from reductions in A&E attendances and hospital admissions.

- Strong emphasis on developing digital services so that within five years, all patients will have the right to access GP consultations via telephone or online.

- Commitment to fully integrated community-based health care. This will involve developing multidisciplinary teams, including GPs, pharmacists, district nurses, and allied health professionals working across primary care and hospital sites.

3 – Mental Health and Learning Disabilities

- Create a more comprehensive service system – particularly for those seeking help in crisis – with a single point of access for adults and children and 24/7 support with appropriate responses across NHS 111, ambulance and A&E services.

- Significant expansion of services for children and young people, including the creation of 'mental health support teams' in schools.

- Two new commitments: (i) Create a comprehensive offer for children and young people, from birth to age 25, with a view to tackling problems with transitions of care. (ii) Redesign core community mental health services by 2023/24, reinforcing components such as psychological therapies, physical health care and employment support, as well as introducing personalised care and restoring substance misuse support within NHS mental health services.

- Strong focus on improving care for people with learning disabilities and autism, including increasing access to support for children and young people with an autism diagnosis, developing new models of care to provide care closer to home and investing in intensive, crisis and forensic community support. The aim is that, by 2023/24, in-patient provision for people with learning difficulties or autism will have reduced to less than half of the 2015 level.

ACUTE SERVICES

1 – Urgent and Emergency Care

- Roll out of GP-led Urgent Treatment Centres (UTCs) across the country by 2020, which will include access to some simple diagnostics and offer appointments bookable via NHS 111 for patients who do not need the expertise available at A&E departments.
- All A&E departments to introduce same day emergency care (also known as ambulatory emergency care). This will see some patients admitted from A&E undergo diagnosis and treatment in quick succession so that they can be discharged on the same day, rather than staying in hospital overnight.

2 – Wider Acute Services

- Use technology to fundamentally redesign outpatient services over five years. The aim is to avert up to a third of face-to-face consultations in order to provide a more convenient service for patients, free up staff time and save £1.1 billion a year if appointments were to continue growing at the current rate.

- Reducing delayed discharges from hospital remains a priority. The plan aims to cut the average number of daily delayed transfers of care (DTOC beds) to around 4,000 and maintain that level over the next two years before reducing it further (DTOC beds averaged 4,580 in November 2018).

RESOURCES

1 – Finance and Productivity

- Commitments to return the provider sector to balance by 2020/21 and for all NHS organisations (commissioners and providers) to balance by 2023/24. To achieve this, NHS Improvement will deploy an accelerated turnaround process in the 30 worst financially performing trusts and a new financial recovery fund, initially £1.05 billion, will also be created for trusts in deficit who sign up to their control totals.

- Measures aimed at supporting delivery of integrated care and incentivising system-based working to improve population health. In 2019/20, as part of the process of moving towards system control totals[18], sustainability and transformation partnerships (STPs) and integrated care systems (ICSs) will be given more flexibility to agree financially neutral changes to control totals for individual organisations within their systems.

2 – Workforce

- For nursing, the aim is to reduce the vacancy rate from 11.6 per cent to 5 per cent by 2028. To achieve this, as well as the previously announced 25 per cent increase in nurse undergraduate placements, the plan commits to funding a 25 per cent increase in clinical nursing placements from 2019/20 and an increase of up to 50 per cent from 2020/21.

- Commitment to increase medical school places from 6,000 to 7,500 per year, possibly more. There is also an ambition to shift the balance from specialised

---

[18] Control totals are annual financial targets that must be achieved to unlock access to national funding and other financial benefits.

to generalist roles in line with the needs of patients with multiple long-term conditions.

- The long-term ambition is to train more staff domestically. In the meantime, it emphasises the need for a continued inflow of international recruits.

3 – Digital

- Digital technology underpins some of the plan's most ambitious patient-facing targets. The NHS app will act as a gateway for people to access services and information; by 2020/21, people will be able to use it to access their care plan and communications from health professionals.

- From 2024, patients will have a new 'right' to access digital primary care services (e.g. online consultations), either via their existing practice or one of the emerging digital-first providers. By the end of the 10-year period covered by the plan, the vision is for people to be increasingly cared for and supported at home using remote monitoring (via wearable devices) and digital tools.

4 – Leadership and Support of Staff

- Range of actions to better support leaders, including doing more themselves to model the style of leadership they wish to see elsewhere in the system, and developing a new 'NHS leadership code' that will enshrine expected cultural values and behaviours.

- Develop and embed cultures of compassion, inclusion and collaboration across the NHS. Specific actions include programmes and interventions to ensure a more diverse leadership cadre, a focus on increasing staff understanding of improvement knowledge and skills, and new pledges to better support senior leaders (including improving the approach to assurance and performance management).

- Do more to support current staff, including increasing investment in CPD, taking steps to promote flexibility and career development, and tackling bullying and harassment.

SYSTEM PRIORITIES

1 – Role of patients and carers

- Fundamental shift required in the way that the NHS works alongside patients and individuals. Highlighting the need to create genuine partnerships between professionals and patients, it commits to training staff to be able to have conversations that help people make the decisions that are right for them. There is also a commitment to increasing support for people to manage their own health, beginning in areas such as diabetes prevention and management.

- Focus on personalisation of care. Referrals to social prescribing schemes[19] will increase, broadening the range of support available, and the roll-out of personal health budgets will be accelerated, so that these are in place for up to 200,000 people by 2023/24. Stronger focus on supporting carers. This includes introducing quality markers for primary care, highlighting best practice in identifying carers and providing them with appropriate support. It also encourages the national roll-out of carers' passports, which enable staff to identify someone as a carer and involve them in the patient's care; and promises a more proactive approach to supporting young carers.

2 – Integrated Care and Population Health

- Shift towards Integrated Care. A new accountability and performance framework will consolidate local performance measures and a new integration index will measure patient and public views about local service integration.

- The move towards a more interconnected NHS will be supported by a 'duty to collaborate' on providers and commissioners, while NHS England and NHS Improvement will continue efforts to streamline their functions.

3 – Prevention and Health Inequalities

- Provision of alcohol care teams in a quarter of hospitals with the highest rate of alcohol dependence-related admissions, and a promise that by 2023/24, NHS-funded tobacco treatment services will be offered to all smokers admitted to hospital. There are also plans to introduce new programmes for specific diseases and conditions, and to scale up existing ones.

- A more concerted and systematic approach to reducing health inequalities', with a promise that action on inequalities will be central to everything that the NHS does. To support this ambition and to ensure that local plans and national programmes are focused on reducing inequalities, specific and measurable goals will be set.

---

[19] Social prescribing, sometimes referred to as community referral, is a means of enabling GPs, nurses and other primary care professionals to refer people to a range of local, non-clinical services.

13.4 Mid-Staffordshire NHS Foundation Trust: The two Francis inquiries

Background

In 2009 the Healthcare Commission (the old NHS regulator) published the findings of an investigation into failings in care at the Mid-Staffordshire NHS Foundation Trust. Focusing on problems at Stafford Hospital, the investigation found widespread failings in care. A local campaign group Cure the NHS, led by Julie Bailey whose mother died at the hospital, campaigned for an inquiry. The previous government ordered two Department of Health investigations and then a secret inquiry led by Robert Francis QC that lacked legal powers and focused on problems at the hospital, not wider failings.

The new coalition government ordered a full legal inquiry under Robert Francis QC who was recognised to have led the first inquiry with sensitivity and care. This inquiry was charged with looking into failings by the various bodies and regulators that are supposed to prevent problems in care persisting.

One of the most worrying things about the scandal was that the Trust had managed to achieve coveted "foundation status" whilst the problems were ongoing. This process required the support of the local Department of Health (known as Strategic Health Authorities), the NHS financial regulator Monitor and the Department of Health directly, including a government minister.

The Healthcare Commission report (March 2009)

The report highlighted a series of failures, particularly in A&E, AMU and on some medical and surgical wards. Those concerns related to:

- Poor nursing standards
- Lack of effective management systems for emergencies
- Failure to identify and act on high mortality rates for patients admitted as emergencies
- A Board detached from day-to-day reality of patient care
- Failure by the Board to develop an open culture and to challenge current practice despite information pointing to obvious problems.

The report qualified the care received by patients as "appalling" and mentioned that this likely led to hundreds of unnecessary deaths. In March 2009, the Chairman was asked to resign by Monitor and the Chief Executive of the Trust resigned in order to avoid being suspended and investigated by the Board.

In December 2009, a review published by the Royal College of Surgeons qualified the Trust as "dysfunctional" and "frankly dangerous".

The first Francis inquiry (2010)

The first inquiry was designed to identify key failures and make recommendations. Led by Robert Francis QC, it identified a "bullying culture, target focused in which the needs of the patients were ignored", and "an appalling failure at all levels".

Key failures identified included:

Board failures
- The Board buried its head in the sand, failed to appreciate the enormity of the issues, reacted too slowly and generally downplayed the significance of many of the issues identified.
- The Board responded to the Healthcare Commission report with denial. It showed no lack of urgency to resolve the issues raised.
- The CEO had concluded that high mortality rates were due to coding issues.
- The Board set out to gain foundation status in order to improve the Trust's governance, making it its number 1 priority. This likely distracted it from dealing with more basic care-related issues.
- There was much focus on finances (the Trust had been making losses for a few years). To save £10m (8% of its turnover), the Trust set out to make cuts, including removing 150 posts. Wards were badly reorganised (separate floors for surgery and medicine without carrying out any risk assessment), beds were cut and consequently patient care was compromised.
- Poor governance (clinical audit practice underdeveloped, critical incidents not reported or not acted upon, investigation of complaints done by staff from the area which caused the problem in the first place (and not seen by the Board)).

Staff-related issues
- Too few consultants and nurses.
- Constant change of management, leading to lack of leadership.
- Doctors isolated from managers, the Board and each other.
- Some key individuals were unsafe.
- Lack of attention to patient dignity (incontinent patients left in degrading conditions, patients left inadequately dressed in full public view, patients handled badly – sometimes by unskilled staff – causing pain and distress, rudeness, hostility, failure to refer to patients by name).
- Poor communication (lack of compassion and sensitivity, lack of information about patients' condition and care, lack of involvement of patients in decisions. Friends and family often ignored, failure to listen and reluctance to give information, staff not communicating well with each other, wrong information provided to patients and relatives).
- Poor diagnosis and management (slow or premature discharge of patients, discharge from A&E without appropriate diagnosis or management, poor record keeping, poor or delayed diagnosis).
- Buzzers left unanswered

Cultural issues
- Patients concerned about insisting on proper care for fear of upsetting staff or of reprisals.
- Staff distracted by their own mobile phones.
- Staff not focused on basics (litter left on the floor, alcohol gel not replenished and therefore not used).
- Low staff morale.

The second Francis inquiry (2013)

The second inquiry focused on commissioning, supervision and regulation of the hospital, querying particularly why such serious issues were not identified earlier and acted upon sooner. The inquiry highlighted the following issues:

- Too much focus on finance, figures, targets and not enough on patient care (recent reforms emphasise outcomes rather than targets) and failure to put patients first.
- Criticism of nursing training and lack of compassion in nursing profession.
- Lack of accountability – attitude that it's someone else's problem e.g. managers vs. clinicians vs. Board vs. politicians. Key will be new Friends and Family test (at Mid Staffs only ¼ of staff would have recommended the hospital).
- Defensiveness, secrecy and complacency – focusing relentlessly on positives and closing eyes to negatives, i.e. poor standards.
- Doctors failed to speak up for patients.
- PCTs and SHAs had blind trust in the hospital's management and accepted their reassurance without further checks.
- Monitor and CQC did not challenge enough.
- The Royal College of Nursing was not supportive enough of its members when they raised concerns.
- Department of Health too remote.
- GPs did not raise concerns until after the issues came to light.

Amongst the 290 recommendations the report made, here are some of the key ones:
- There should be more focus on compassion and caring in nursing recruitment, training and education.
- Patient safety should be the number 1 priority in both medical and nursing training and education.
- Individuals and organisations would have a duty to speak up (the government is in fact considering the possibility of criminal prosecution for staff who don't).
- Quality accounts should be published in a common format and made public.
- The profession of healthcare assistants should be regulated.
- For the elderly, one person should be in charge of individual patient care.
- The RCN should be either a royal college or a trade union.
- Patient involvement must be increased.
- Structural change is not the answer.

The government's response (27 March 2013)

- Duty of candour to be placed on NHS boards to be honest about mistakes.
- Consideration being given to making individual doctors and nurses criminally responsible for covering up errors.
- New ratings system for hospitals and care homes based on Ofsted scheme used in schools.
- Posts of Chief Inspector of hospitals and care homes to be created; and possibly primary care.
- Nurses to spend up to a year working as a healthcare assistant so they get experience providing basic care such as washing and dressing.
- Managers who fail in their jobs to be barred from holding such positions in the future.
- Code of conduct and minimum training standards for healthcare assistants, but not full registration scheme as recommended by inquiry.
- Tough rules to be drawn up to allow Trusts to be put into administration when basic standards are not met unless problems can be resolved quickly.
- Department of Health civil servants to be forced to spend time on the front line of the NHS.
- Prof. Don Berwick was asked to set up an inquiry into "making harm a zero reality in the NHS" – National Advisory Panel on the Safety of Patients.

13.5 Duty of Candour

The new statutory duty of candour was introduced for NHS bodies in England (trusts, foundation trusts and special health authorities) on 27 November 2014, and applied to all other care providers registered with CQC from 1 April 2015. The obligations associated with the statutory duty of candour are contained in regulation 20 of The Health and Social Care Act 2008 (Regulated Activities) Regulations 2014. The key principles are:

1. Care organisations have a general duty to act in an open and transparent way in relation to care provided to patients. This means that an open and honest culture must exist throughout an organisation.

2. The statutory duty applies to organisations, not individuals, though it is clear from CQC guidance that it is expected that an organisation's staff cooperate with it to ensure the obligation is met.

3. As soon as is reasonably practicable after a notifiable patient safety incident occurs, the organisation must tell the patient (or their representative) about it in person.

4. The organisation has to give the patient a full explanation of what is known at the time, including what further inquiries will be carried out. Organisations must also provide an apology and keep a written record of the notification to the patient.

5. If the patient cannot be contacted or refuses to engage, a written record is to be kept of attempts to contact or to speak to him/her.

6. A notifiable patient safety incident has a specific statutory meaning: any unintended or unexpected incident that occurred in respect of a service user during the provision of a regulated activity that, in the reasonable opinion of a health care professional, could result in, or appears to have resulted in:

    - the death of the service user, where the death relates directly to the incident rather than to the natural course of the service user's illness or underlying condition, or
    - severe harm, moderate harm, or prolonged psychological harm to the service user.

    'Severe harm' means a permanent lessening of bodily, sensory, motor, physiologic or intellectual functions, including removal of the wrong limb or organ or brain damage, that is related directly to the incident and not related to the natural course of the service user's illness or underlying condition.

'Moderate harm' means harm that requires a moderate increase in treatment (that is, an un-planned return to surgery, an unplanned re-admission, a prolonged episode of care, extra time in hospital or as an outpatient, cancelling of treatment, or transfer to another treatment area (such as intensive care); and significant, but not permanent, harm.

7. There is a statutory duty to provide reasonable support to the patient. Reasonable support could be providing an interpreter to ensure discussions are understood, or giving emotional support to the patient following a notifiable patient safety incident.

Once the patient has been told in person about the notifiable patient safety incident, the organisation must provide the patient with a written note of the discussion, and copies of correspondence must be kept.

13.6 Revalidation

The origins of revalidation

The idea of revalidation arose many years ago at the result of several medical scandals. Its aim is to ensure doctors' fitness to practise. Revalidation aims to protect patients from poorly performing doctors, promote good medical practice and increase public confidence in doctors.

Under the original proposals, doctors would have submitted records of appraisals, including personal development plans and feedback. They would also have submitted CPD records. Based on that evidence the GMC would have decided whether to revalidate a doctor or insist on further action.

The 5th Shipman Report and suspension of revalidation

Following the Shipman affair, in which Dr Shipman, a GP, had single-handedly murdered hundreds of his patients over a number of years without being suspected or detected, an inquiry was conducted by Dame Janet Smith into the various components of the scandal. This included an inquiry into the role of the GMC, which resulted in the so-called 5th Shipman Report. The report essentially criticised the GMC for looking after doctors more than after patients and for not taking reasonable steps to protect patients by revalidating doctors properly. It also highlighted the poor sharing of information on doctors' performance between the professional, educational and regulatory bodies. The GMC's role was also criticised, particularly the fact that it sets the rules, investigates doctors and passes judgement on their actions.

When the GMC was criticised for letting Harold Shipman kill hundreds of victims unnoticed, it defended itself by presenting revalidation as the answer to the problem.

The Shipman case mainly concerned a failure by the NHS to audit Shipman's activities in a number of areas including:

- Cremation forms (and a second signature more or less applied without checks).
- A high mortality rate amongst his patients (all of whom were elderly and whose deaths were simply dismissed as unlucky or natural).
- A discrepancy in the prescription of diamorphine and other controlled drugs (all the more bizarre since Shipman had already been suspended by the GMC for stealing drugs in the 1970s).

It was established that Shipman was well liked by colleagues and patients, and therefore would have passed appraisals with flying colours. He also kept up to date and would have had no problem being revalidated on the basis of those two criteria only. As a result the GMC had no choice but to suspend revalidation (before it was fully introduced) and to go back to the drawing board.

Better doctors, safer patients (14 July 2006)

On 14 July 2006, Professor Sir Liam Donaldson, the Chief Medical Officer (CMO), published his review into the regulation of the medical profession. The report was designed to address the criticism raised against the GMC in the 5th Shipman Report issued by Dame Janet Smith.

The main recommendations in the *Good Doctors, Safer Patients* document included:

- The creation of unambiguous, operationalised standards for generic and specialist practice to give a clear, universal definition of a "good doctor" and to allow patients, employers and doctors themselves to have a shared understanding of what is expected of doctors. These standards would be incorporated into the contracts of doctors.

- Devolution of some of the powers of the GMC, as statutory regulator, to the local level. This would be accomplished through the creation of a network of trained and accredited General Medical Council affiliates.

- The creation of an independent tribunal in order to adjudicate on fitness to practise matters – the GMC would focus on the assessment and investigation of cases.

- A renewed focus on the assessment, rehabilitation and supervision of doctors with performance problems where these problems are not borne of malice.

- Greater public and patient involvement – to ensure public and patients work with GMC affiliates in making decisions around fitness to practise, and with medical Royal Colleges in the process of recertification.

- A new twin-track system of revalidation – relicensing for all doctors and recertification for those on the specialist and GP registers.

These principles were adopted in the government's White Paper on professional regulation, *Trust Assurance and Safety – The Regulation of Health Professionals in the 21st Century* in February 2007.

Renewed attempt at introducing revalidation (2009)

Following on from the July 2006 *Good Doctors, Safer Patients* report by Liam Donaldson, an extensive consultation period was undertaken, resulting in a new document *Medical Revalidation: Principles and Next Steps* issued by a group led by Liam Donaldson.

Revalidation would be made up of two strands: Relicensing and Recertification.

Relicensing
The relicensing process was designed to ensure that doctors practise in line with the standards set out by the GMC. It consists mainly of annual local appraisals relying upon multi-source feedback.

One problem was that the NHS appraisal process as it stood was inadequate. In addition, it would also be inappropriate to impose a unique appraisal system when there is such diversity of work, settings and practices within the system. As a result, it was concluded that the appraisal process may indeed be designed by each employer for its own needs but that it should contain one standardised module agreed by the GMC. This would ensure that the process is appropriate for each doctor and simultaneously fulfils the GMC's criteria.

Relicensing was formally introduced in November 2009.

Recertification

The principles used to recertify doctors were to be set out by the appropriate Royal Colleges and specialist associations. The evaluation process would, of course, vary between specialties and may involve simulators, etc. It was recommended that "high-stakes" tests should be avoided, which effectively means that doctors won't be assessed with just one test but across a series of tests.

Because relicensing deals with the general standards whilst recertification deals with the specialist standards, both would be combined in one single recommendation to the GMC as to whether a doctor should be revalidated or not.

Recertification was meant to be introduced in 2010 but implementation was delayed until late 2012 as Royal Colleges struggled to arrive at a consensus on how to recertify their members. The main hurdles to implementation were:

- Logistics: There were 150,000 doctors who needed to be revalidated every 5 years. Trusts and the GMC would need to make sure that the revalidation steps were timed appropriately to avoid bottle-necks. There may be a challenge with doctors who come in and out of the system (e.g. maternity, fellowships, any non-clinical practice, etc).

- Method: Because the process will be driven locally, it would be challenging to ensure that it is applied consistently.

- Connecting: There would be a need to ensure that the revalidation process was linked to other processes of quality assurance, patient safety and quality improvement (e.g. audits, patient questionnaires, etc.).

- Information: Appraisals and recertification would require the ready availability of a large amount of data. Care would need to be taken that the data is available.

- Cultural: Doctors would need to buy into the process and should not view it as a threat. Simultaneously, patients should not view the process as a smoke screen.

Revalidation at last! (Late 2012)

The process

Revalidation started on 3 December 2012 and the majority of licensed doctors in the UK are expected to revalidate for the first time by March 2016. Revalidation consists of regular appraisals with the employer, based on the GMC's *Good Medical Practice*.

- Licensed doctors are required to link to a Responsible Officer.

- Licensed doctors need to maintain a portfolio of supporting information drawn from their practice which demonstrates how they are continuing to meet the principles and values set out in the Good Medical Practice Framework for appraisal and revalidation.

- Licensed doctors are expected to participate in a process of annual appraisal based on their portfolio of supporting information.

- The Responsible Officer makes a recommendation to the GMC about a doctor's fitness to practise, normally every 5 years. The recommendation is based on the outcome of a licensed doctor's annual appraisals over the course of 5 years, combined with information drawn from the clinical governance system of the organisation in which the licensed doctor works.

- The GMC's decision to revalidate a licensed doctor is informed by the Responsible Officer's recommendation.

The portfolio

The portfolio needs to contain the following information, which should be discussed at the appraisal:

- General information such as personal details, scope of work, record of annual appraisals, personal development plans and their review, statement on probity and health.

- CPD record.

- Review of your practice including quality improvement activities such as clinical audit, review of clinical outcomes or case review; and description of significant events.

- Feedback on your practice including colleague and patient feedback, as well as a review of complaints and compliments.

Pros of revalidation

- Formalises practices which may have been done on an ad-hoc basis previously.

- Ensures compliance with some basic requirements and provides focus for the appraisal process.

Cons of revalidation

- Will not stop another Shipman.

- Senior clinicians may see it as their way to fulfil their management responsibilities and may consequently not ensure proper management of individuals at other times of the year.

- Runs the risk of identifying underperformance only at the "once-a-year appraisal point", i.e. in some cases too late.

- The process may require information that Trusts do not hold (e.g. for surgeons, individual results).

- It takes time to gather the information. Various organisations estimate that doctors will need approximately 2 hours a week to comply with requirements. This could prove tricky if Trusts cut down the time doctors can spend on non-clinical activity in order to maintain efficiency and profitability.

13.7 The appraisal process

Overview

An appraisal is essentially a constructive discussion with a senior colleague during which a doctor reflects on his performance and considers how he may be able to improve his practice. The appraisal process forms an important part of the revalidation process.

During the appraisal, the doctor is being given feedback on his performance, which will have been provided in advance by members of his team. Any development needs can then be assessed and solutions can be implemented to remedy any issues. Although it is not their primary goal, appraisals can be particularly useful in spotting early signs of underperformance so that it can be addressed at an early stage before developing into an irremediable problem.

As well as looking at past performance, the appraisal process helps the doctor identify development needs in relation to his career aims.

Personal development plans (PDP)

As an outcome of the appraisal, key development objectives for the following year and subsequent years should be set. These objectives may cover any aspect of the appraisal such as personal development needs, training goals and organisational issues, continuous medical education (CME) and CPD.

What is the difference between appraisals and assessments?

The difference can be summarised as follows:

- An assessment is essentially checking whether your practice matches a set of defined criteria set out in some kind of curriculum (e.g. test or exam, including the workplace-based assessments).

- An appraisal, however, places the focus on identifying learning needs with a view to optimising your career and personal development.

A more simplistic view is: an assessment is similar to an exam, whereas an appraisal is a constructive discussion on future development needs.

13.8 The NHS in Wales, Scotland and Northern Ireland

There are virtually no questions being asked on political issues in interviews in Wales, Scotland and Northern Ireland. I have set out below basic information which will give an indication of the key features of the health system in each country.

Wales

The reorganisation of NHS Wales, which came into effect on 1 October 2009, created single local health organisations that are responsible for delivering all healthcare services within a geographical area, rather than the Trust and Local Health Board system that existed previously. The reorganisation abolished the internal market.

There are seven Health Boards. In Wales, healthcare funding is still based on block contracts between Welsh commissioners and the relevant providers. Funding to hospitals from Welsh commissioners is therefore based on historical activity and funding levels as a guide for the expected number of treatments over the coming year. Clinical activities are not funded on the basis of actual activities provided. Instead, an overall figure of anticipated activity is agreed in advance between the commissioner and the provider.

The Health and Social Services budget is £6 billion: 40% of the Welsh Assembly's total budget. From 1 April 2007 the NHS prescription charge was abolished for people in Wales.

Scotland

The Scottish Government Health Directorate (SGHD) has responsibility for NHS Scotland as well as the development and implementation of community health policy. The SGHD undertakes the central management of NHS Scotland and heads a Management Executive that oversees the activity of the 14 area NHS Boards.

The roles of the Health Boards include strategic leadership and performance management of the entire local NHS system in their areas and assurance that services are delivered safely, effectively and cost-efficiently. The 14 NHS Boards are ultimately responsible for the commissioning, provision and management of the full range of health services in an area including hospitals and General Practice.

Payment to hospitals is on a block contract basis. Like Wales, Scotland offers free prescriptions to its residents. The budget for NHS Scotland is £11 billion, just over one-third of the Scottish government's annual budget.

Northern Ireland

In Northern Ireland the National Health Service is referred to as HSC or Health and Social Care. Just like the other NHS it is free at the point of delivery but in Northern Ireland it also provides social care services such as home care services, family and children's services, day care services and social work services.

The Department of Health, Social Services and Public Safety has overall authority for health and social care services. Services are commissioned by the Health and Social Care Board and provided by five Health and Social Care Trusts – Belfast, the largest of the five, South Eastern, Southern, Northern and Western.

The Health and Social Care Board sits between the Department and Trusts and is responsible for commissioning services, managing resources and performance improvement. Inside the Board there are Local Commissioning Groups (LCGs) focusing on the planning and resourcing of services. The LCGs cover the same geographical areas as the five Health and Social Care Trusts.

The budget for the Department of Health, Social Services and Public Safety is £4 billion: 40% of the Northern Ireland Executive's annual budget.

14 Body language and dress code

Much has been written about body language and you may find various statistics quoted, such as body language represents about 60% of your communication.

Whilst there is no doubt that body language is important in helping you make a good impression, one should not forget that, ultimately, your body language is a reflection of your confidence and that confidence is not something that you acquire solely by smiling politely and moving your arms properly. There is a danger that a candidate may concentrate heavily on his/her appearance at the expense of building content and structure into his/her answers.

As you gain more and more confidence through your preparation, your body language will change and will open up naturally. I would therefore recommend that you do not worry about it until you are well advanced in your preparation.

The key rules of body language

If your interview consists of several stations of 10 minutes each, you will need to build a rapport and make a good impression quickly. Here are a few key rules that you will need to follow:

Eye contact
This is the most crucial part of your relationship with the interviewers as far as body language is concerned. No one will be interested in listening to someone who is not looking straight at them so make sure that you maintain good eye contact with whoever is asking you the question. Occasionally look at the other person too so that they feel included.

Seat position
If you are sitting behind a table, make sure that you are not too close or too far from the table. If you are too close, you will have difficulty relaxing and also your elbows will be forced to rest on the table. The interviewers would feel that you are invading their space and may be forced to back away from you. If you are too far from the table, you will either start slouching in your seat, giving the impression that you don't really care, or you will lean forward reaching for the table. Not only will you get lower back pains, but you will also appear very casual. A good distance is about 10cm from the table so that your arms can rest on the table comfortably with the elbows remaining outside the table and not on it.

Arm positions
Many candidates find it comfortable to have their hands under the table. This gives an impression of timidity and of trying to hide behind the furniture. You need to project an image of quiet confidence and having your hands on the table will help you achieve that.

Hand movements
It is perfectly acceptable to move your hands if it is part of your personality. Don't force yourself if it doesn't come naturally to you though. If you are someone whose hands tend to move naturally, make sure that you contain that movement to the space in front of you and no higher than chest level; otherwise your hand movements will start obstructing your face.

Dress code

There are hundreds of ways in which you can make a good impression with your dress code and, in a way, it would be patronising to impose a general way of dressing. What matters is that you are comfortable in your clothes and that they are fit for the purpose of a professional meeting. It often helps to mirror the dress code of those interviewing you (generally conservative).

There are some general rules that will make a difference in the way in which people perceive you though:

Dress to frame your face
The focal point should be your face; therefore you want to frame your face by wearing darker colours on the outside and lighter colours on the inside. For men, this will mean a shirt of light tone and for women a light-coloured blouse. This should be complemented by a dark-toned suit.

Look neat
If you wear a beard, make sure you trim it. If you wear make-up, don't overdo it. Clip your nails, tidy your hair, and make sure none of it obstructs your face. I know it sounds obvious but you would be surprised.

Avoid distracting features
Continuing on the theme of your face being the focal point, avoid any features or accessories which may draw the eye to the wrong places. In particular: no sequins (they make wonderful disco balls when light reflects off them), no brooches, no ribbons, poppies, or other symbols which are either too big or too bright in colour.

Small items of jewellery may be okay providing they do not steal the limelight away from you and do not draw the attention away from your face.

PRACTICAL INTERVIEW STATIONS

15 Communication station

Communication/role-play stations have become increasingly common at interviews in many specialties. They are based on realistic scenarios, with the patient being played either by an interviewer or a professional actor. Role plays are designed to test your communication skills more than your clinical skills – though inevitably a relevant clinical knowledge is essential to perform well – and the marking schemes reflect this, i.e. if you have excellent communication skills but talk rubbish, you will not pass the station.

The marking scheme

A variety of marking schemes have been used for communication/ role-play stations in the past. Typically, two interviewers would assess the candidate on a range of communication criteria. Each criterion is marked independently on a scale from 0 to 4, with 0 = Poor and 4 = Excellent and comprehensive. All marks are then added across all criteria and both interviewers to form the final mark. In some cases, the actor is also asked for their opinion on their feelings about the candidate from the point of view of the patient. A typical marking scheme would look as follows:

	Interviewer 1	Interviewer 2	Total mark
Setting the scene	0 to 4	0 to 4	0 to 8
Listening abilities	0 to 4	0 to 4	0 to 8
Verbal communication	0 to 4	0 to 4	0 to 8
Non-verbal communication	0 to 4	0 to 4	0 to 8
Content	0 to 4	0 to 4	0 to 8
Overall impression	0 to 4	0 to 4	0 to 8
Total	**Max score 24**	**Max score 24**	**Max score 48**

Criteria will vary in their wording and in the manner in which they are grouped (e.g. in some deaneries/specialties, verbal and non-verbal communication are marked together) but the expectations and overall criteria are the same.

Timing and preparation time

The actual consultation time will vary between 8 and 20 minutes depending on the deanery and specialty.

In most role-play stations you will be given some time to prepare. This varies from a few minutes to up to 20 minutes. Make sure you make the best use of that preparation time to read the brief given to you and the patient's history so that

- you do not miss any crucial information during the consultation; and

- you do not waste time during the consultation asking the patient about information that you have been told you already know. Some actors may have been instructed to act angry if they have to repeat information which is in the brief.

Running the role play

In order to score well, you will need to ensure that you address the following:

Understanding of the impact of the environment on the consultation
In some role plays, the room will be set up with the doctor's and the patient's chairs in a position which may not be ideal to build a rapport with the patient. If you feel it appropriate, you may want to move your chair and the patient's chair so that they are at an appropriate distance. If there is a table, you should ensure that you are not sitting across the table from the patient but that you are only separated by a corner of the table. Explain you have passed your bleep to someone else and do not expect to be disturbed during the consultation/meeting.

Introduction
Greet the patient by name if the brief gives it to you. Introduce yourself by name. Shake their hand if the patient is willing to accept and take the patient to the seat reserved for them (some actors may be instructed to remain standing until you invite them to sit down. If the situation warrants it, ask if they have come accompanied and if they want their relative or friend to sit in on the conversation. If you have been given a task (e.g. breaking bad news), then start by giving an overview of how the conversation will run, how long for and say that you will end with a clear, agreed management plan. If you or the department has caused the patient some harm, it is important to start with an apology.

Encourage the patient to tell you about the problem using open questions such as "What can I do for you today?" If the patient has been recalled to see you for a specific purpose, you can start more directly by explaining the reason for the recall.

Listening & Empathy
When discussing the issue at stake with the patient, allow the patient time to talk. Do not interrupt them unless you feel that you really need to. There are times when one needs to learn to keep quiet.

Be attentive to what they are telling you. The actor will have been primed to drop certain clues into the conversation, either voluntarily or taking one of your questions as a cue. In role play, candidates are often so obsessed with what they should do next that they sometimes forget to listen to the patient.

Throughout the conversation, observe the patient's behaviour. Listening does not necessarily mean hearing their words. You can pick up a lot of information by observing their body language. An awkward body language may give you clues about something that the patient is not telling you or is feeling embarrassed or scared about.

If the patient is silent or uncommunicative, encourage them by asking open questions. If the patient is distressed, it may also prove valuable to simply allow the situation to remain silent for a while if talking does not help. This may help them regain their composure.

History taking, diagnosis and clinical information
Ask all questions relevant to the scenario and explain any necessary points. Try not to ask for information that you should already know from the brief as you may irritate the patient. However, if you feel the need to confirm some information with the patient, either because the brief is ambiguous or the patient has contradicted information that you were given, then you may double-check.

Explain your diagnosis to the patient (including any differentials). Use words which are appropriate for the patient. Ensure that the patient understands what you are explaining; if necessary ask them to confirm their understanding by repeating in their own words what they have understood and by using questions such as "Is there anything that you do not understand?" or "Is there anything that you would like me to clarify?" If appropriate, explain using different methods or media (some spare paper may be made available to you).

Do not go into overdrive on the clinical section of your consultation at the expense of everything else. Clinical management accounts for, at most, 20% of the overall mark.

Holistic & psychosocial needs
The interviewers will be testing your ability to identify the various needs of the patient and how you address them during the consultation. Consider the physical aspects of the problem, but also the psychological and social sides. How is the patient coping? What is the impact on their family? What support is available to them? Make sure that you elicit the patient's ideas, concerns and expectations.

Body language
The manner in which you attempt to build a rapport with the patient and the appropriateness of your body language play an important role in your success at handling any role play. Make sure that you keep an open posture (no crossed arms),

avoid being above or too close to them, lean slightly forward to show empathy when required, nod in the right places and, most important of all, maintain good eye contact with the patient to maintain that crucial rapport. Eye contact will also enable you to read the patient's emotions and possible discomfort, which could provide valuable clues. If they look like they may cry, a hand on their hand or shoulder may be appropriate or you could pass them some tissues.

The unexpected

Some role plays are fairly mainstream (i.e. they attempt to replicate a normal consultation or scenario without any particular surprises). Others have twists and turns, which may catch you off-guard. This may include a patient who suddenly becomes irate, a patient who suddenly withdraws, refuses to say any more and looks down, a patient who cannot speak a word of English, or a patient who takes you onto a completely unexpected path.

When this happens, you must always remember that it is a game, i.e. this was planned. Rather than give up, try to remain calm and see how you can help the situation along. If the patient has walked out, see if you can get them back by using a more diplomatic approach. If the patient is not talking, don't just look at the examiners in despair; see if you can re-engage. If the patient throws you off-guard by mentioning issues that you were not expecting, don't look flustered or stunned. If you are, then ask the patient to elaborate on what they have just said; it will give you some time to regain your composure (and might help you score some listening points). If a patient is angry, slow down the speed of your conversation and become quieter; hopefully they will match you.

Ending the consultation

Role plays can be conducted in different manners. In some cases, the interviewers will let you know when you have 2 minutes left, but in many cases they won't. The first you will hear from them is the sound of a bell and a "thank you – you can move to the next station" grunt. Make sure that you keep track of time so that, if possible, you can draw the conversation to a natural close. Most marking schemes will include an allowance for your conclusion so make sure you get there. If you feel that you are likely to run out of time because you went off on a tangent or allowed the patient a bit too much space, then make a quick assessment of the situation and determine whether it is worth sacrificing 1 mark for not having a conclusion but gaining several more marks by addressing several other important issues instead.

Towards the end of the consultation, you should summarise to the patient what action is being proposed and what they have agreed to. You should also explain whether follow-up will be required and when. Thank them for coming and escort them to the door.

If your role play is over 20 minutes and you have finished before the end of the official period, ask yourself whether you have forgotten any important aspects and cover these as necessary. If not, then don't be afraid of terminating the exercise a few minutes early. It is better to end on a confident note than to waffle on for 2 minutes to kill time.

Examples of role plays

Topics will obviously vary per specialty but here are some examples of role plays which were part of recent interviews. I have stated the specialties in which they were asked, but some of these could be asked in many specialties.

- O&G: Explain to a patient who can only speak very little English that she has an ectopic pregnancy and needs an urgent procedure. The patient does not understand what you mean and is begging you to save the baby.

- Diabetes: A recently diagnosed patient explains that she does not trust her GP to have made the correct diagnosis about her diabetes. She is a single mother who makes ends meet by driving a taxi part-time.

- A&E: You diagnosed a patient with dyspepsia. He later died following an MI. You are now being confronted by an angry widow.

- Oncology & General Surgery: A patient was recently diagnosed with breast cancer. She is now refusing treatment and would like to opt for homeopathy instead.

- Dermatology: You recently reassured a patient that their mole was non-malignant. The patient returns to you, having sought a second opinion from another hospital, and accuses you of incompetence. A preliminary investigation showed that you had mixed up two biopsy results with two patients of the same name.

- Psychiatry: An old lady with dementia who lives in a care home presents to A&E with bruises. The A&E consultant leaves you on your own with the patient.

- Ophthalmology: Explain to an educated patient what glaucoma is. Once you have provided your explanation they express extreme fear at the prospect of becoming blind.

- CMT/Surgery in general: You are meeting the relative of an elderly woman, who is expressing concerns at the news she has read on MRSA in the NHS. Your hospital has a very good record and very low morbidity/mortality rate associated with MRSA but the relative has just spotted that the consultant's tie was brushing against all patients.

- Surgery: Break the news to a male patient that he has colorectal cancer. He is a fit athlete.

- Paediatrics: You requested a CT scan for a young patient. The radiologist has refused to do the scan due to the excessive radiation the child would be exposed to. The parents are blaming you for the lack of progress in the management of the patient.

- Paediatrics: Explain to a child what asthma (or diabetes) is.

16 Presentation station

Presentations are a recruitment tool that is on the increase. They have been a common feature at consultant interviews for some time and have recently found their way into ST recruitment.

What is being assessed?

Through your presentation, the interviewers will be assessing:

- Your general presentation skills (confidence, ability to engage an audience, etc.)

- Your ability to communicate your ideas clearly, concisely, using an approach suited to the topic and the audience. This will include marks for the clarity of the slides and their relevance

- The content of the presentation, i.e. the appropriateness and maturity of the content

- Your time management and organisational skills, i.e. your ability to stick to time, to allocate appropriate timing to each of the sections in your talk, etc.

Similar to the communication/role-play station, the marking scheme is likely to score each of the above out of 4, the combined marks of the two assessors forming the candidate's final score.

Preparation time and duration

Presentations generally vary in length between 5 and 10 minutes. Whilst in some specialties you may be asked to prepare a presentation in advance (the details being communicated to you in the invitation letter), in others you are likely to be placed on the spot, with the presentation topic being given to you just 45 minutes before you are due to present. Slides or overheads are usually allowed, though some restrict their number, whilst others require you to speak without visual aids. It is important to clarify the equipment that will be available on the day and then have several failsafe backup options. We have all seen people fail to get their projector working, even at national meetings. Ways to bring digital media include: CD, memory stick, uploaded to the web or emailed to the department. It may be worth copying onto transparencies for an overhead projector or bringing handouts.

Example of topics

Presentation topics are very varied. They generally fall under three different categories:

Generic
- Tell us about yourself
- What can you contribute to this specialty?
- How do you see your career developing, what skills do you have and which would you wish to gain?
- Why do you think you will make a good paediatrician/ orthopaedic surgeon?

Political
- How do current NHS changes impact on this specialty?
- How can this specialty become more efficient?
- How will you make sure that you become a good consultant when working hours are being decreased?

Personal
- Tell us about your hobbies.
- How have your strengths and weaknesses informed your career choice?

Occasionally, you may be asked to talk about some non-work-related topic of your choice. This has led to candidates making presentations on topics as varied as:
- How to teach cricket to 10-year-old children
- How to fly a helicopter
- The history of chocolate
- Silver hallmarking

Essentially, presentations can be regarded as extended interview questions, which you have 10 minutes rather than 2 minutes to answer. In that sense similar principles apply with regard to the need to structure the information around three or four themes or ideas and the need to make the information memorable by giving examples. There is nothing worse than a presentation which is too theoretical. Relate it to your audience.

Key principles

There are a few rules that you will need to remember during your preparation.

Keep the number of slides to a minimum
The rule of thumb is to have no more than 1 slide per 90 seconds of talk. Therefore, a 10 minute presentation should contain no more than six or seven slides. If your talk is organised around four central ideas (as it should be), then you would only need 1 slide for each plus an introduction and a summary slide, making six slides in total.

Keep the slides short and simple – the 4 by 4 rule

Never forget that the slides are there to support your presentation and help your audience. They are not there to replace your notes because you can't be bothered to learn your talk. If the slides are too busy then the interviewers will struggle to read them and to listen to you at the same time. The best slides are those which stick to the main principles and allow the audience to focus their attention on the candidate. As a general rule, you should have no more than 4 bullet points, each with no more than 4 words (this is called the 4 by 4 rule).

You should also ensure that any text written on the slides is large enough to be seen from a distance. You may want to ask beforehand whether the slides will be projected onto a screen (even if through an overhead projector) or simply read from a laptop. Whatever method they choose, your slides should be readable from a laptop screen which is 3 metres away. If they are not then there is either too much text or the font size is too small. Generally have high contrast between text and background (e.g. black on white or white/yellow on dark blue).

Vary your slides and make them accessible

Always think whether there is a more interesting way of representing your message than through a standard bullet point. For example, if I want to convey that there are four issues that the NHS is focusing on currently, I could simply list them as bullet points, for example:

- Efficiency
- Training
- Quality
- Profitability.

Alternatively, I could convey the same with four pictures on my slide:

- Efficiency: a picture of an organised or a chaotic unit
- Training: a picture of a ward round, or of a lecture
- Quality: a picture of a "tick"
- Profitability: a picture of a money bag or a pound sign.

Pictures, graphics and other means of visual representation are often very powerful and, in the meantime, your audience does not spend hours trying to decipher whole lines of text written in font size 8 in a desperate bid to make it all fit onto the page. Some of the best presentations I have seen included one candidate who used pictures only, no words, and a candidate who simply opted to use no visual aids. The effect it had was that the interviewers could then pay full attention to his talk. It is worth checking whether slides are essential (i.e. whether their quality will be judged) or whether they are just accepted, as this may give you ideas for how to make your talk more interesting. Try to avoid being too flashy or using complicated animations, transitions and movies, even if you are an expert. The interviewers are likely to use an old version of Windows, an old version of Microsoft Office and a slow computer.

Prepare a good speech, rehearse and take your time to deliver it

At the risk of stating the obvious, you must make sure that you rehearse your presentation many times so that you know it well, even without any visual aids. You should rehearse the presentation at least four times, two of which should be under time pressure, ideally in front of a scary panel!

Your speech, and not the slides, should be the main focus of the presentation. If you have prepared your visual aids properly, there should still be plenty of information that you need to add to your presentation verbally. Your speech will bring colour to your presentation, will bring personal reflection onto your ideas and will guide the audience through their journey of discovery.

As a rule, you should allow approximately 160 words per minute of speech. If you have to speak too quickly to get to the end of the presentation within the allocated time then you have too much information. Go back to the drawing board and see if all the information that you are presenting is relevant. If it isn't relevant or if it confuses matters then take it out. Be ruthless: the simpler the presentation, the better. Often the problem is linked to a lack of proper structure or the wrong structure. See if you can reorganise the information using different headings. Having more complex slides also increases the risk of you being out of synch with them and that is confusing for the audience.

Prepare some notes

During the presentation itself, it is preferable that you do not use notes. The danger of using notes is that you will inevitably be tempted to look at them. Also, reading them will make you sound wooden. However, you should bring a set with you just in case you have a memory gap. Make sure that they are hidden from you in your jacket pocket and that they are in a suitably small size (i.e. postcard size rather than A4) so that you can just pull them out of your pocket if need be without looking too flustered.

Watch your voice & delivery
- Your voice must be confident and normally loud.
- Avoid dropping your voice at the end of your sentences.
- Pause briefly between each slide. You might know your topic well but your audience will need time to keep up with you.
- Find good ways to link the slides.
- Do not rush your delivery.

Watch your body language
- Smile! Even a nervous smile is more endearing than a depressed or terrorised look.
- Adopt a natural stance. This means having your feet 25cm apart with your knees very slightly bent. Relax your shoulders.
- Be aware of your natural habits. Some people have a tendency to play with loose change in their pockets, to sway from one foot to the other, to play with

a pen or their watch strap. You must be able to identify those habits and squash them before someone on the panel finds them irritating.
- Keep your hands in front of your belly. You can move them but not in an exaggerated fashion.

How to prepare

A common problem with presentations is the lack of clarity and simplicity in the message that the candidates want to convey. This results in complicated and confused slides, which then translates into a poor delivery. To perform well, you will first need to make sure that you have your story in the right order. Once you have looked at the topic, start talking about it in your head or aloud and see what comes out. Once you have perfected the story, you will be much better able to identify the key points that form its structure and its logic. Those points will form the backbone of your presentation and will dictate your slides. If you commit your thoughts too early to paper or to slides, you will lose flexibility. You will be reluctant to change the order of your slides or review the entire structure of your talk for fear of having wasted your preparation time. Not committing your talk to paper too early will enable you to adopt a totally different approach without having to rewrite a lot of material. Try to reframe from another's point of view. Try taking a system (helicopter) view or see the topic from the point of view of a commissioner or a patient or the panel themselves. What would be important or interesting for each of these stakeholders?

17 Group discussion station

Group discussions are gradually being introduced in several specialties, though they are still fairly uncommon outside General Practice recruitment.

Format of the group discussion

Group discussions typically last 20 minutes. There will usually be four people in each group, sitting around a table, with each being assessed by an external observer. In some cases, there may be just one observer for two candidates. The team is given a brief shortly before the session commences and, at the agreed time, the required discussion needs to start.

There are two main types of group discussions:

- *Normal discussion*
  The group is given a general topic of discussion and has to debate the issues involved. In many cases, the discussion is based on a simple 2-line brief such as an ethical issue. In other cases, the information provided is more comprehensive and may include, for example, a letter of complaint addressed to your consultant or extracts from patient notes. In other, more complex group discussions, the candidates may actually be given different pieces of information; for example, one candidate may have a summary of the notes, another candidate will be given a complaint letter, another an abstract from a report, etc.

- *Role-play group discussion*
  In this type of group discussion, each candidate is allocated a different role. One candidate may be playing the SHO, another candidate a senior nurse, another candidate the GP and the fourth candidate a social worker. The roles obviously depend on the type of scenario given.

What the assessors are looking for

Much as it is tempting to show off your knowledge of the topic being discussed, this is only one of the areas that the assessors will be looking for. Indeed, if they wanted to test your knowledge, they would either ask you a direct question in a normal interview setting or ask you to do a presentation.

The assessors will, however, be far more interested in the manner in which you interact with the rest of the group. This can be very complex to assess when people can have such diverse personalities. Some candidates will be natural leaders and they may well feel at ease driving the conversation. Other candidates may be good facilitators, i.e. they get on well with most people and are able to keep the peace. Others still may contribute much to the team by generating content and ideas but could not lead or facilitate.

What the interviewers will be looking at therefore is a general pattern of behaviour that fits well within a team and your interaction with others, whatever your personality. This will include

- Your general contribution to the discussion (which can include active listening, support of others and encouraging opinions from the quieter members)
- Your problem-solving abilities
- Your general interaction with others including your body language and the appropriateness of your behaviour (empathy, sensitivity, situation awareness)
- Your ability to cope with the challenges of working within a team (e.g. pushy colleagues, uncooperative people, quiet people, etc.)
- Clarity of communication and assertiveness if necessary
- Your ability to influence/negotiate with people, i.e. to rally people to your point of view without making them feel coerced.

Dealing with difficulties within the group

Going round in circles
There may be a time when the conversation has ceased to be productive and the team has either gone off on a tangent or is caught in a vicious circle. In such cases, you would score marks for enabling the team to get back on track by gently reminding everyone of the original goal and pointing out in a non-threatening manner that you all got lost. Bring the focus back to the patient, to avoid making things confrontational.

Awkward silences
The team may have reached a natural break in the discussion, or it may be that no one dares speak in case they say something stupid. If this happens, you should encourage the team to summarise the discussion so far, to set out the main themes that could be discussed and then to ensure that the points are dealt with systematically. If the conversation has ended because all points were discussed, then finish the exercise early; do not go on waffling until the bell rings.

Overbearing colleagues
Some talk a lot because they are extroverts; extroverts tend to think while they talk and may actually change their opinion 180 degrees very quickly. Others may talk a lot due to nerves. There will always been one in the group who will have misunderstood the point of the exercise, thinking that he will look clever by showing off his knowledge of the topic being discussed. Such people can do themselves much damage but can also take you down with them if you are not careful. Indeed, by

occupying the space and monopolising the time available, they do not allow you the platform that you need to show off your own team-playing skills.

If you are that person, then make sure you allow others to have a say and encourage them. If you are faced with such a colleague, the best way to handle the situation with different strategies is:

- Asking others what they feel about what this person has said
- Asking for a break in the discussions so that you can summarise the points made so far
- Directly letting the colleague know that it would be useful for others to comment so that you can get different perspectives on the problem.

Silent colleague

Some are silent because they are introverts, doing lots of thinking in their heads and then waiting to give a considered answer. Ask them directly and wait for 7-8 seconds for a reply. Others may just feel uncomfortable with the role-play technique, be anxious as it is part of the interview or just not know the answer.

By themselves silent colleagues may not feel like a threat because they give you the floor. But in fact, if you ignore them and do not encourage them, you may be marked down. Pay attention to those around so that you can spot them.

If you are that person then you will need to make an effort to participate, at least by encouraging others. No silent candidate will score anything. If you want to demonstrate that you are a good listener then you will need to make sure that you demonstrate this not just by listening but also by summarising the points made so far and helping the team move forward.

If you are faced with a silent colleague, try to encourage them to participate by asking for their opinion at an appropriate moment. If they refuse to be involved, then do not force them as it would count against you but demonstrate at least that you are making an effort.

USEFUL

RESOURCES

18 Action and power words

The vocabulary and turns of phrase that you use at an interview will make a big difference to the way in which your answers are perceived by the interviewers and the confidence and maturity that you exude.

Part of your maturity and confidence will come from the spontaneity and fluency of your answers, both of which can be addressed through practice, but much of it will come from using words which convey your meaning powerfully.

The impact of action and power words

Consider these sentences:
- I would be happy to play a role in teaching.
- I have been lucky to be involved in audit over the past two years.
- I have had the opportunity to be involved in research.
- My consultant has asked me to be involved in research.
- I have been part of a team which developed guidelines on <xxx>.

None of these really convey a strong sense of commitment and enthusiasm. At an interview, saying such sentences would be okay in small doses, but if repeated too often they will give the feeling that you are not in control of your career and that you are adopting a passive stance.

- "I would be happy" basically means "Ask me nicely and I would do it".
- "I have been lucky" conveys that you did not choose to get involved but that you rely on others to give you opportunities.
- "I have had the opportunity" makes you rely on the chance that someone (or fate) will create an opportunity where you can get involved.
- "My consultant has asked me" may be what actually happened but again it makes you look dependent and not in charge of your destiny.
- "I have been part of a team" may be okay as an introduction if you then go on to talk about yourself but does not convey your own role and, as such, runs the risk that you may be selling the achievement of the team rather than your own.

There are tighter, more assertive and more powerful ways of selling yourself by using what is termed "power" or "action" words. For example:
- "I have <u>developed a strong interest</u> in teaching and am very <u>keen to take on</u> a more prominent role over the next few years."

- "I have <u>played a key role</u> in managing audit projects from data collection to presentation stage."
- "I <u>discussed with my consultant</u> a number of research opportunities, following which I <u>embarked on a project</u> which looked at <xxx>"
- "I <u>reviewed</u> our morbidity rate following procedure <xxx> and, as a result, I <u>worked closely</u> with two of my colleagues to introduce new guidelines on <yyy>."

These power words will help you convey your meaning in a more distinct manner and will make a lot of difference to your final mark.

List of action and power words

Here is a list of over 500 power words that you can use to increase the strength of your answers. These can be used not only in formal interview questions but also in role play and group discussions.

Abbreviated	Abolished	Abridged	Absolved
Absorbed	Accelerated	Acclimated	Accompanied
Achieved	Acquired	Acted	Activated
Actuated	Adapted	Added	Addressed
Adhered	Adjusted	Administered	Admitted
Adopted	Advanced	Advertised	Advised
Advocated	Affected	Aided	Aired
Allocated	Altered	Amended	Amplified
Analysed	Answered	Anticipated	Applied
Appointed	Appraised	Approached	Approved
Arbitrated	Arranged	Articulated	Ascertained
Asked	Assembled	Assessed	Assigned
Assisted	Assumed	Attained	Attracted
Audited	Augmented	Authored	Authorised
Awarded	Balanced	Began	Benchmarked
Benefited	Bid	Billed	Blocked
Boosted	Borrowed	Bought	Branded
Bridged	Broadened	Brought	Budgeted
Built	Calculated	Canvassed	Captured
Cared	Cast	Catalogued	Categorised
Centralised	Chaired	Challenged	Changed
Channelled	Charged	Charted	Checked
Circulated	Clarified	Classified	Cleared
Closed	Coached	Co-authored	Collaborated

Collected	Combined	Commissioned	Committed
Communicated	compared	Compiled	Completed
Complied	Composed	Computed	Conceived
Conceptualised	Condensed	Conducted	Conserved
Consolidated	Constructed	Consulted	Contacted
Contributed	Controlled	Converted	Conveyed
Convinced	Coordinated	Copyrighted	Corrected
Corresponded	Counselled	Created	Critiqued
Cultivated	Customised	Cut	Dealt
Debated	Debugged	Decentralised	Decreased
Deferred	Defined	Delegated	Delivered
Demonstrated	Depreciated	Described	Designated
Designed	Detected	Determined	Developed
Devised	Diagnosed	Directed	Discovered
Dispatched	Dissembled	Distinguished	Distributed
Diversified	Divested	Documented	Doubled
Drove	Earned	Eased	Edited
Educated	Effected	Elicited	Eliminated
Emphasised	Empowered	Enabled	Encouraged
Endorsed	Enforced	Engaged	Engineered
Enhanced	Enlarged	Enlisted	Enriched
Ensured	Escalated	Established	Estimated
Evaluated	Examined	Exceeded	Exchanged
Executed	Exempted	Expanded	Expedited
Experienced	Explained	Explored	Exposed
Extended	Extracted	Fabricated	Facilitated
Fashioned	Fielded	Financed	Fired
Flagged	Focused	Forecasted	Formalised
Formatted	Formed	Formulated	Fortified
Founded	Fulfilled	Furnished	Furthered
Gained	Gathered	Gauged	Generated
Governed	Graded	Granted	Greeted
Grouped	Guided	Handled	Headed
Helped	Hired	Hosted	Identified
Ignited	Illuminated	Illustrated	Impacted
Implemented	Improved	Improvised	Inaugurated
Incorporated	Increased	Incurred	Individualised

Indoctrinated	Induced	Influenced	Initiated
Innovated	Inquired	Inspected	Inspired
Installed	Instigated	Instilled	Instituted
Instructed	Insured	Integrated	Interacted
Interpreted	Intervened	Interviewed	Introduced
Invented	Inventoried	Invested	Investigated
Invited	Involved	Isolated	Issued
Joined	Judged	Justified	Kept
Launched	Lectured	Led	Lightened
Liquidated	Litigated	Lobbied	Localised
Located	Logged	Maintained	Managed
Manufactured	Mapped	Marketed	Maximised
Measured	Mediated	Mentored	Merchandised
Merged	Minimised	Modelled	Moderated
Modernised	Modified	Monitored	Motivated
Moved	Multiplied	Named	Narrated
Navigated	Negotiated	Netted	Noticed
Nourished	Nursed	Nurtured	Observed
Obtained	Offered	Opened	Operated
Orchestrated	Ordered	Organised	Oriented
Originated	Overhauled	Oversaw	Participated
Patented	Patterned	Performed	Persuaded
Phased	Photographed	Pinpointed	Pioneered
Placed	Planned	Polled	Posted
Prepared	Presented	Preserved	Presided
Prevented	Processed	Procured	Produced
Proficient	Profiled	Programmed	Projected
Promoted	Prompted	Proposed	Prospected
Proved	Provided	Publicised	Published
Purchased	Pursued	Qualified	Quantified
Quoted	Raised	Ranked	Rated
Received	Recognised	Recommended	Reconciled
Recorded	Recovered	Recruited	Rectified
Redesigned	Reduced	Referred	Refined
Regained	Registered	Regulated	Rehabilitated
Reinforced	Reinstated	Rejected	Remedied
Remodelled	Renegotiated	Reorganised	Repaired

Replaced	Reported	Represented	Rescued
Researched	Resolved	Responded	Restored
Restructured	Resulted	Retained	Retrieved
Revamped	Revealed	Reversed	Reviewed
Revised	Revitalised	Rewarded	Safeguarded
Salvaged	Saved	Scheduled	Screened
Secured	Segmented	Selected	Separated
Served	Serviced	Settled	Shaped
Shortened	Shrank	Signed	Simplified
Simulated	Sold	Solicited	Solved
Spearheaded	Specialised	Specified	Speculated
Spoke	Spread	Stabilised	Staffed
Staged	Standardised	Steered	Stimulated
Strategised	Streamlined	Strengthened	Stressed
Structured	Studied	Submitted	Substantiated
Substituted	Suggested	Superseded	Supervised
Supplied	Supported	Surpassed	Surveyed
Synchronised	Systematised	Tabulated	Tailored
Targeted	Taught	Tested	Tightened
Took	Traced	Tracked	Traded
Trained	Transacted	Transcribed	Transferred
Transformed	Translated	Transmitted	Transported
Treated	Tripled	Troubleshot	Tutored
Uncovered	Underlined	Undertook	Unearthed
Unified	United	Updated	Upgraded
Urged	Used	Utilised	Validated
Valued	Verbalised	Verified	Viewed
Visited	Visualised	Voiced	Volunteered
Weathered	Weighed	Welcomed	Widened
Withstood	Witnessed	Won	Worked
Wrote	Yielded		

19 Reference websites

DH (Department of Health)
www.doh.gov.uk

NHS Choices
www.nhs.uk

GMC (General Medical Council)
www.gmc-uk.org

MMC (Modernising Medical Careers)
www.mmc.nhs.uk

NICE (National Institute for Health and Clinical Excellence)
www.nice.org.uk

ROYAL COLLEGES & FACULTIES

Royal College of Physicians
www.rcplondon.ac.uk

Royal College of Physicians of Edinburgh
www.rcpe.ac.uk

Royal College of Physicians and Surgeons of Glasgow
www.rcpsg.ac.uk

Royal College of Surgeons of England
www.rcseng.ac.uk

Royal College of Surgeons of Edinburgh
www.rcsed.ac.uk

Royal College of Anaesthetists
www.rcoa.ac.uk

Royal College of Obstetricians and Gynaecologists
www.rcog.org.uk

Royal College of Paediatrics and Child Health
www.rcpch.ac.uk

Royal College of Pathologists
www.rcpath.org

Royal College of Psychiatrists
www.rcpsych.ac.uk

Royal College of Radiologists
www.rcr.ac.uk

Royal College of Emergency Medicine
https://www.rcem.ac.uk/

Faculty of Occupational Medicine
www.facoccmed.ac.uk

Faculty of Public Health
www.fph.org.uk

DEANERIES

NORTH

North East (including North Cumbria)
https://madeinheene.hee.nhs.uk/

North West
https://www.nwpgmd.nhs.uk/

Yorkshire and the Humber
https://www.yorksandhumberdeanery.nhs.uk/

MIDLANDS AND EAST

East Midlands
https://www.eastmidlandsdeanery.nhs.uk/

West Midlands
https://www.westmidlandsdeanery.nhs.uk/

East of England
https://heeoe.hee.nhs.uk/

SOUTH

Kent, Surrey and Sussex
https://ksseducation.hee.nhs.uk/

South West: Peninsula Region
http://www.peninsuladeanery.nhs.uk/

South West: Severn Region
http://www.severndeanery.nhs.uk/

Thames Valley
http://www.oxforddeanery.nhs.uk/

Wessex
http://www.wessexdeanery.nhs.uk/

LONDON
https://www.lpmde.ac.uk/

20 Key documents

Good Medical Practice (2013)
Available from the GMC's website at www.gmc-uk.org

Raising and acting on concerns about patient safety (2012)
Available from the GMC's website at www.gmc-uk.org

Confidentiality (2009)
Available from the GMC's website at www.gmc-uk.org

Consent: patients and doctors making decisions together (2008)
Available from the GMC's website at www.gmc-uk.org

0-18 years: guidance for all doctors
Available from the GMC's website at www.gmc-uk.org

Mental Capacity Act 2005
Available from the Office of Public Sector Information
www.opsi.gov.uk/ACTS/acts2005/ukpga_20050009_en_1

This document is complex to read (legal jargon and with a formal legal format) so I would recommend that you read it only if you have an interest in these issues and a few hours to spare! Otherwise the summary provided in section 11.8 will be more than enough.

FULL INDEX OF QUESTIONS AND ISSUES

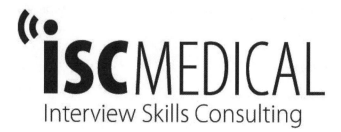

ISC Medical is the UK leader in the provision of courses for medical interviews and personal development.

We provide a wide range of courses for candidates applying to CT / ST / Registrar posts, including:

- **CT/ ST Registrar interviews (1 day)**
- **Teach the Teacher / Train the Trainer (2 days)**
- **Leadership and Management (2 days)**
- **Advanced Communication Skills (2 days)**
- **Assertiveness and Influencing (1 day)**
- **Public Speaking (1 day)**
- **Coaching and Mentoring (1 day)**

10% discount on all courses

Use disco

WW